I0269837

BECOMING VEGAN IS ONE OF THE MOST IMPORTANT AND DIRECT CHANGE WE CAN MAKE TO SAVE THE PLANET AND ITS SPECIES.

PHOTOGRAPHY
by NAZLI DEVELI

DESIGN
by STUDIO AURORA

EDITOR
STELLA NILSSON

All rights reserved. First Printing 2018, Copyright by Nazlı Develi. This book or any portion thereof may not be reproduced or used in any manner whatsoever without the express written permission of the publisher except for the use of brief quotations in a book review.

Hardcover Edition - Revised & Expanded Second Printing, March 2022
ISBN 9781736374276

Independently published by Nazlı Develi

For information about permission to reproduce selections from this book, write to hello@gurmevegan.com
www.gurmevegan.com
www.greenandawake.com

GREEN & AWAKE

GOURMET VEGAN

100 ELEVATED EVERYDAY GOURMET RECIPES

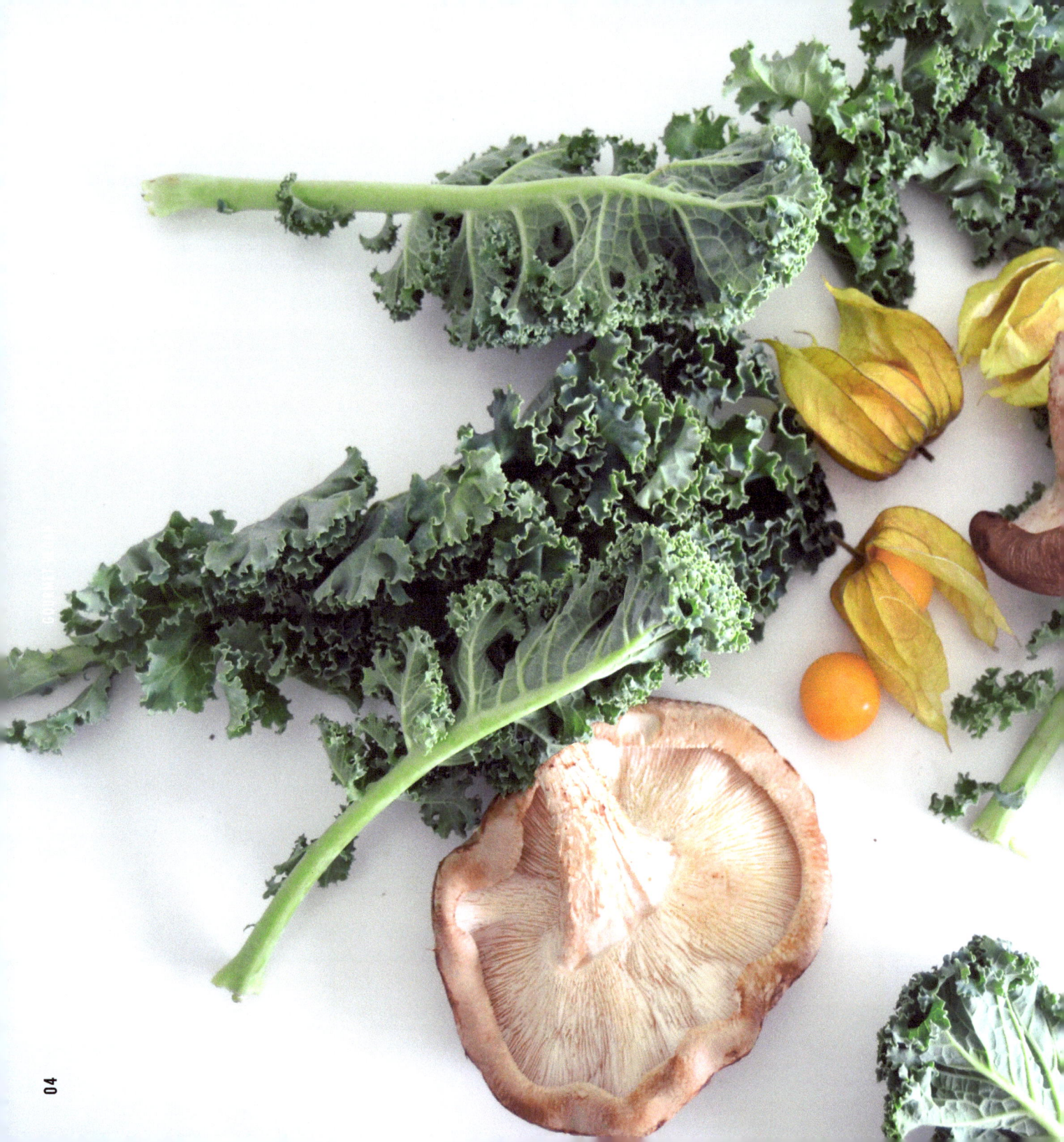

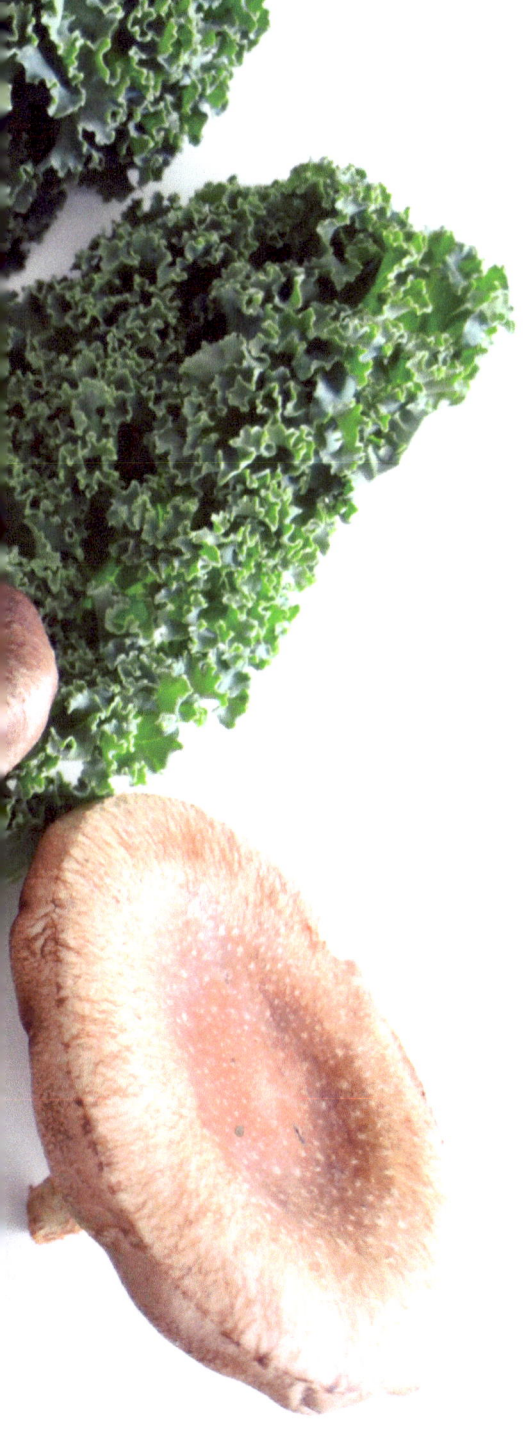

CONTENT

Introduction	06
First Bites	09
Soups	47
Salad Bowls	59
Mains	103
Sweets	153
Index	204
About the Author	207

INTRODUCTION

I spent my childhood in the kitchen with my chef grandfather. After many corporate experiences and learning processes in my life journey, I had a deep spiritual experience in a pachamama ceremony. In 2014, when I questioned the abnormality of an animal-eating diet, was introduced to the concept of "veganism" and I had a quick transition shortly after awakening.

In this book, I combined the knowledge I have aquired for years with my intuitive side and tried perfecting the art of plant-based cooking.

This book helps people become better in the kitchen with a minimalist approach to cooking. It allows me to use my food science knowledge for good. The amount of equipment, with easy steps involved, and the time we spend in the kitchen to a minimum so we can focus what's important. It's about simple gourmet food that is easy to prepare and still fun and satisfying to eat.

I invite you to find out positive effects of Green & Awake food on to the mental and physical impacts sizing the journey of your life.

I see sharing and spreading experiences as a social responsibility towards future generations. When we look into the world, insatiable ego, ambition, endless wars, persecution of other creatures are always due to negative energy.

The person who eats the body of a dead animal is fed with the negative energy of the animal that is created by it's artificial and involuntary farm life.

A person spreads this negative energy to the others and it leads to a life that has been in vain with the bad karma that it creates.

On the way to individual improvement, to nourish vegan is imperative.
Vegan nourishing also encircles other spiritual sides of the foods such as foods having a higher vibration which are healthier rather than the dead ingredients.

Also there is more about the spiritual side; thoughts of the person who makes the meal, affects the quality of the food. Being in touch with natural - not fabricated - ingredients during the cooking process, feeling the nature and it's enormous offerings, makes people happier than unnatural ingredients.

In this book, I have prepared elevated everyday gourmet recipes that you will enjoy more and more when you stop eating animals.

The state of your mind while you are cooking, directly affects the quality of food. It is possible to transform every meal into a medical joy by conscious cooking.

Each color, sound, thought and emotion have its own vibration. We're all made of vibrational energy and connected spiritually by the energy. We need to consume the energy in various forms such as water, air and food.

We do not need only vitamins or minerals. It is the aura of the food and what kind of spirit joins when it is brought together. In short, while eating, we take our thoughts or the emotions and thoughts of others.

Food Designer, Chef & Author

GOURMET VEGAN

FIRST BITES

MACADAMIA CHEESE

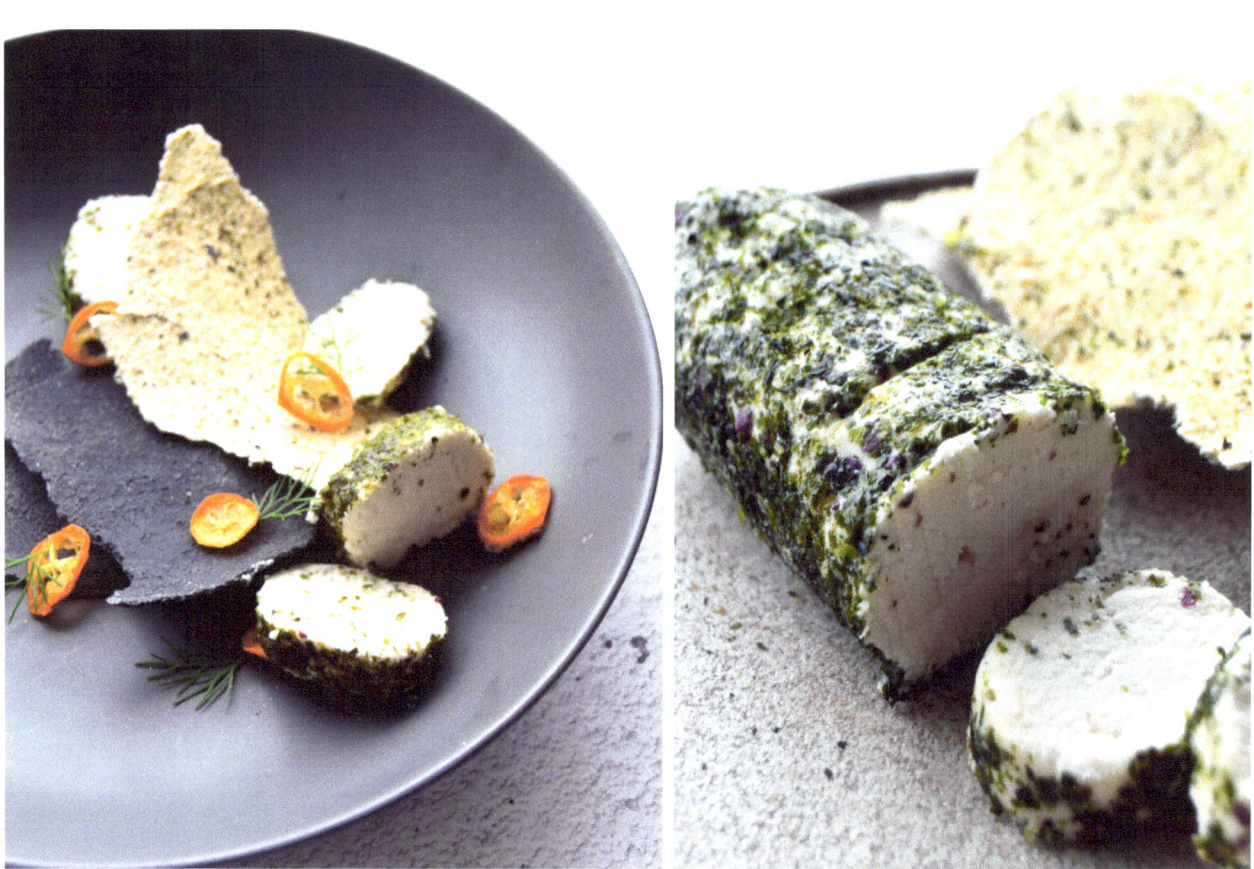

Nuts contain levels of phytic acid equal to or higher than those of grains. When we ferment the nuts, phytates are eliminated. Soaking nuts makes the food more digestible.

Time - 50 minutes
Serves - 6

Ingredients

220 g raw macadamia nuts
4 g acidophilus probiotic
1/3 cup filtered water
2 tbsp nutritional yeast
2 tbsp lemon juice
1/4 tsp sea salt
1/2 bunch fresh dill or seaweed powder

1. Place the nuts in a jar. Cover with filtered warm water and close the jar. Let it rest in the room at least 1 hour. Then place in the fridge for 6 hours. This process will activate the nuts and also yields a neutral nut flavor.
2. Set 6 tablespoons water from the soaked nuts aside. Strain and rise nuts. Place nuts and 6 tablespoons water into the food processor. Mix on high speed until silky smooth. If you are using probiotic powder then dissolve it in a little water.
3. Then transfer into the food processor. Mix well. Transfer nut mixture into a nut milk bag. Gather up the ends to create a ball. Wrap the ends and squeeze out any excess moisture.
4. Place cheese in the dehydrator at 30° C for about 20-24 hours to let it ferment.
House with an average temperature of 25-30º C for 24 hours.
5. Once the fermentation time is up, open the cheesecloth and observe your nut cheese very carefully. You will probably notice that a yellowish crust has formed on top. That is totally normal. The inside of the nut cheese should be spongy. If there is pink or bluish spots, it indicates the presence of mold; throw away the cheese and restart. If everything is ok, transfer cheese from its cloth to a bowl and stir in nutritional yeast, garlic, lemon juice and salt.
6. At this point you could add in other flavors whatever you like. If you like a stronger cheese flavor, add a bit more nutritional yeast. Form a log or ball on a piece of parchment paper and place in the fridge for overnight.
7. Last step is rolling in a salty herby mixture. On a flat surface, spread out fresh dill or seaweed powder and sprinkle on some salt. Take your cheese and give it a good roll in the herbs.
8. Place in the fridge at least 3 days to age the your cheese.
If you like a softer cheese, you can use cashews instead of macadamia nuts, or a mix of both nuts. In that case, you will need less than ½ cup of water, because cashews are creamier to blend.

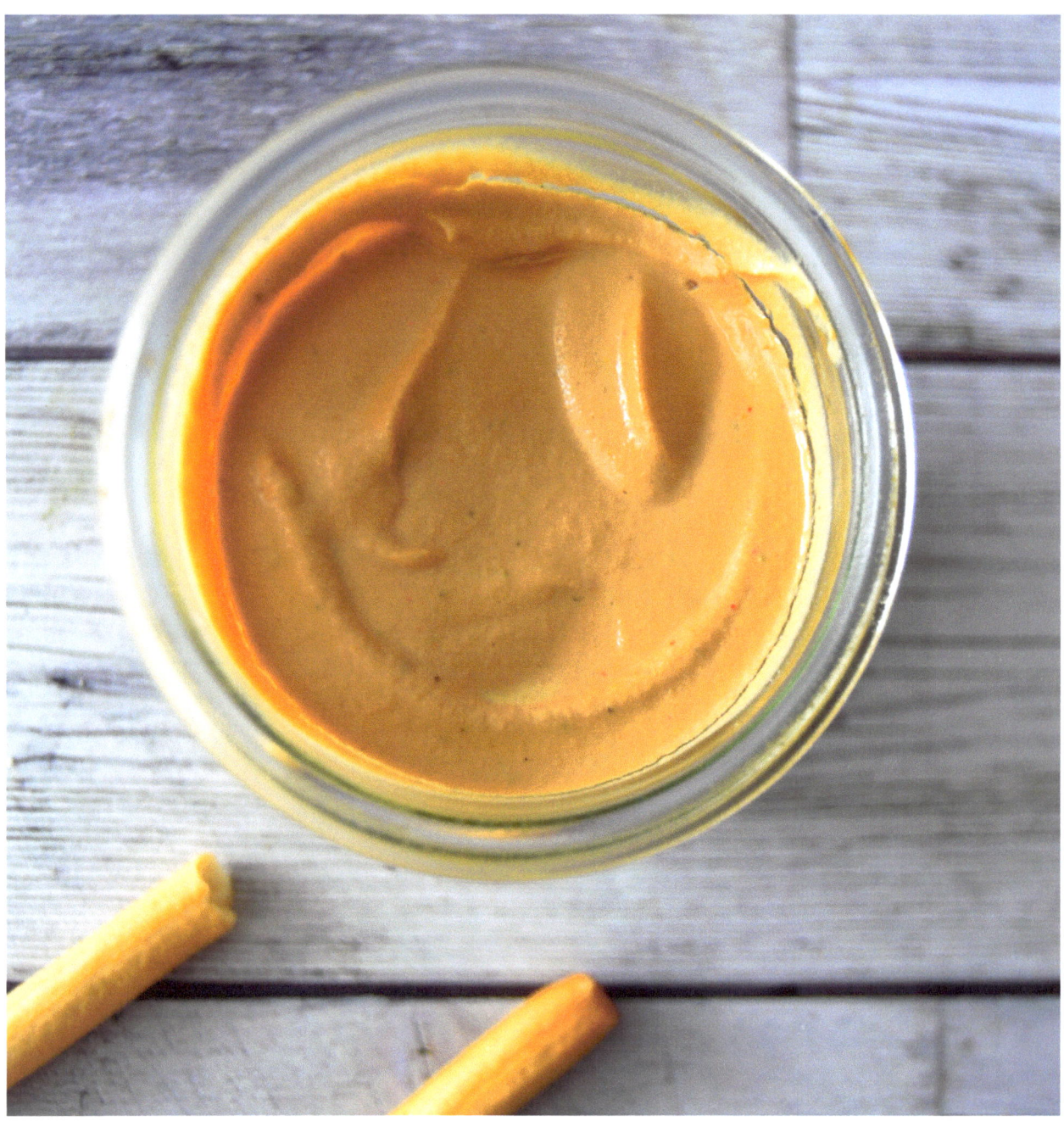

SPREADABLE CULTURED CHEDDAR

This cultured vegan cheddar cashew cream cheese is incredibly simple to make and packed with all the beloved tanginess of the real thing. It is also spreadable, perfect to serve with sandwiches or as an appetizer.

Time - 20 minutes
Serves - 6-8

Ingredients

200 g raw cashews soaked
250 ml rejuvelac (see below)
Juice of 1/2 lemon
1 tsp apple cider vinegar
1 tbsp tomato paste
1 tsp miso
1 tsp paprika
1 tsp smoke liquid
1/2 tsp turmeric powder
2 tbsp nutritional yeast

For the rejuvelac

1/2 cup raw quinoa
2 cups water

1. Start making rejuvelac first. Wash and drain your quinoa, place into a glass jar. Cover with filtered water.
2. Let your jar sit at room temperature away from direct sunlight for 6 to 8 hours.
3. Then drain the water. Rinse the grains a couple times. Drain water again and cover the top of jar with a cheesecloth or very thinly kitchen towel.
4. Let the grains sit at room temperature until sprouted, it takes about 1 to 2 days. Keep the grains from drying out by rinsing and draining them 2 to 4 times a day.
5. When your grains have started to sprout, rinse them one more time and drain well.
6. Fill your jar with fresh water again. Let it ferment for 2 to 3 days.
7. When mixture started to ferment, you will see bubbles in the water. And then the water will seem cloudy. This is totally normal. when the mixture reach up to this, it is ready.
8. Strain the liquid into a new jar and keep in the refrigerator. It is ready to use for cultured cheese.
9. If you need more liquid, add more water in the jar to create second batch. It takes 1-2 days. Repeat the process for this.
10. To make cultured cheddar, Blend soaked cashews and aquafaba in a high speed blender until smooth.
11. Strain mixture to remove large particles. Then transfer mixture to your blender again. Add lemon juice, tomato paste, turmeric, paprika, nutritional yeast, miso and then pulse in the blender to combine them well. Add apple cider vinegar and smoke liquid and blend again until silky smooth. Taste and add salt as you need. If the mixture is very thick, you can add some water (about 50 ml) and mix well afterwards.
12. Pour mixture into a glass jar. Refrigerate 3 hours before using.

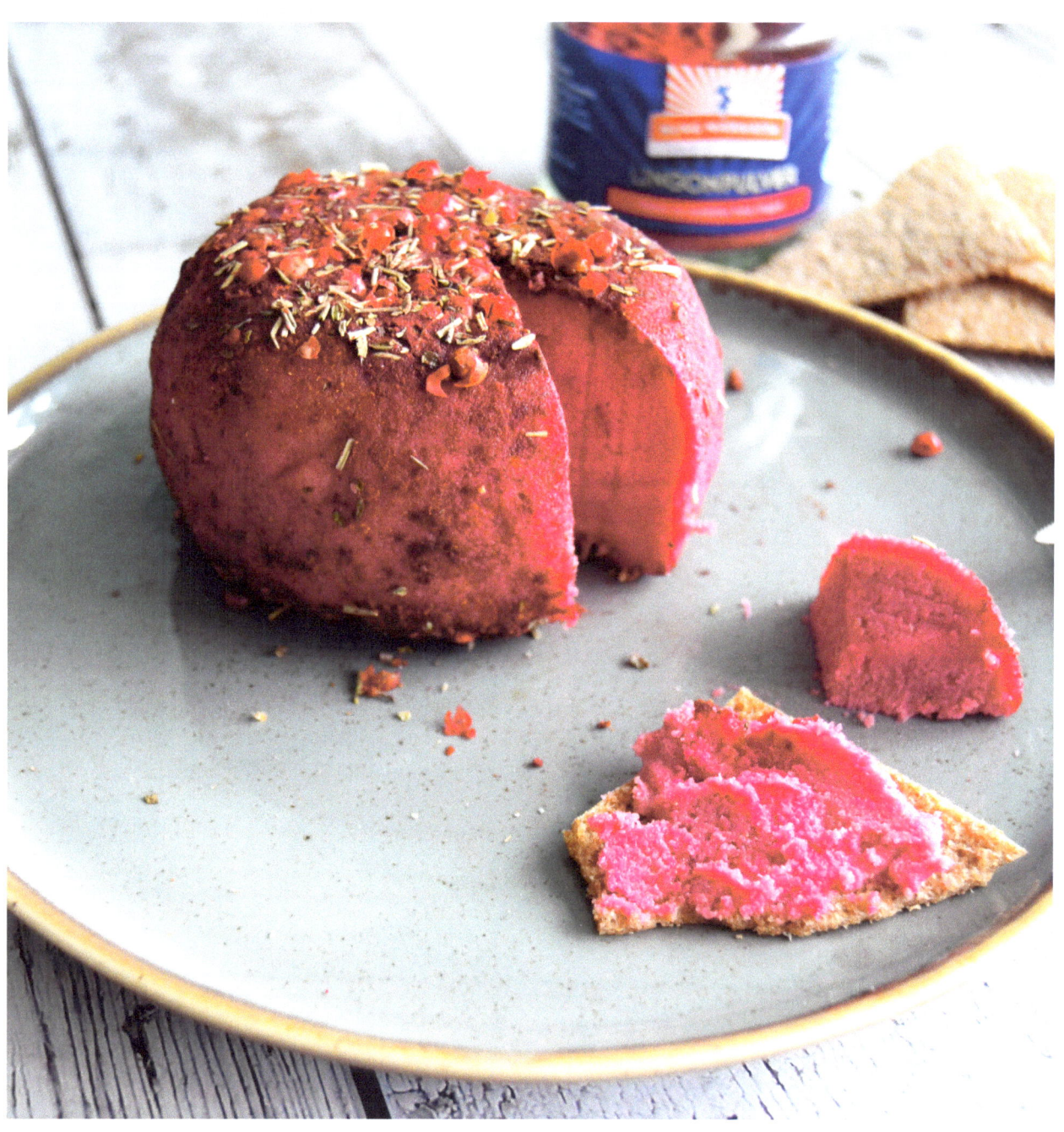

PINK ALMOND CHEESE

Time - 50 minutes
Serves - 6

Ingredients

220 g raw almonds
2 probiotic capsules
3 tbsp filtered water
1 tbsp nutritional yeast
75 ml lemon juice
1/2 tsp salt
1 small beetroot
4 tbsp dried rosemary for coating
1 tbsp lingonberry powder for coating (optional)

1. Place soaked rinsed nuts into food processor, add probiotic powder and water. Mix on high speed until smooth.
Transfer nut mixture into a nut milk bag. Gather up the ends to create a ball.
2. Wrap the ends and squeeze out any excess moisture.
Place cheese in the dehydrator at 30° C for 24 hours to let it ferment. (House with an average temperature of 25-30°C for 24 hours.)
3. Once the fermentation time is up, open the cheesecloth and observe your nut cheese very carefully. You will probably notice that a yellowish crust has formed on top. That is totally normal.
4. Cook beet until soften. Place into food processor, add a little warm water, blend until puree.
5. Place fermented almond into the food processor, add lemon juice, nutritional yeast, beet puree and salt. Mix on high speed until completely smooth. Form a log or ball on a piece of parchment paper and place in the fridge for 8-10 hours.
6. As you can consume the cheese next day, you can leave it to fermente for a week. The cheese will lost some water day by day, pat it dry with a paper towel if it is too wet and replace the parchment paper with new one. For the 2 next weeks, flip the cheese everyday and change the parchment paper regulary if it becomes wet.
At the end cover with beet, rosemary, pink peppercorns or lingonberry powder. Keep in the refrigerator.

CHEESE FONDUE

Time - 20 min prep + 24 hrs fermentation
Serves - 3-4

Cashew Cream
1 cup cashews soaked
1 cup water
1 capsule probiotic (solgar advanced acidophilus plus works well)

Fondue
1/2 cup vegan white wine
2/3 cup water
1 tbsp maple syrup
3 tbsp gluten-free nutritional yeast
2 tbsp olive oil
1/4 cup tapioca
1/2 tsp onion powder
1 tsp turmeric
1/2 tsp salt
1/2 tsp garlic powder or minced garlic

1. To make cashew cream, drain the soaked cashews and transfer to a high-speed blender.
2. Add the water and blend on high for 20-30 seconds, or until smooth and creamy.
3. Transfer the cashew cream to a clean jar*. Add the powder from one capsule of probiotics and stir it into the cashew cream using a wooden spoon.
4. Cover the jar with plastic film, or with a clean cheese cloth. Let it ferment at room temperature for about 24 hours (or up to 48 hours). The cashew cream is ready once you can see some bubbles and it has a tangy flavor.

5. To make fondue, transfer the fermented cashew cream to a blender and add all of the other ingredients. Blend for 15-20 seconds or until smooth. The fondue will be very liquid, that is normal.
6. Pour the fondue batter into a large saucepan. Heat over medium heat, whisking constantly, until it thickens and starts to get stretchy, about 5 minutes.
You can then serve it immediately, or transfer to a fondue set to keep warm. Dip pieces of bread into the cheese fondue and enjoy!

BIRCHER MUESLI

Time - 15 minutes
Serves -1-2

Ingredients
1 red apple grated
1/2 cup rolled oats
A handful of walnuts or almonds
1 tbsp chia seeds
1 tbsp hemp hearts
1/2 cup coconut yogurt or almond yogurt (alternatively mix silken tofu in the blender with 1 tbsp maple and 1 tbsp lemon juice, then use instead yogurt)
1/4 cup almond milk
1/2 cup fresh raspberries, blueberries or strawberries of your choice
1/4 cup citrus fruits or extra forest fruits of your choice for topping

1. Wash and grate your red apple, add to a mixing bowl.
2. Add the rolled oats over the apples.
3. Then add the walnuts or almonds along with the chia seeds and hemp hearts.
4. Add the coconut yogurt and almond milk, then stir well.
5. Add some fresh fruits of your choice. Mix well.
6. Place in the fridge at least 1-2 hours until thicken.
7. Once thicken, add the preferred toppings, and enjoy!

COCKTAIL PIZZA BITES

Time - 50 minutes

Serves - 4-6

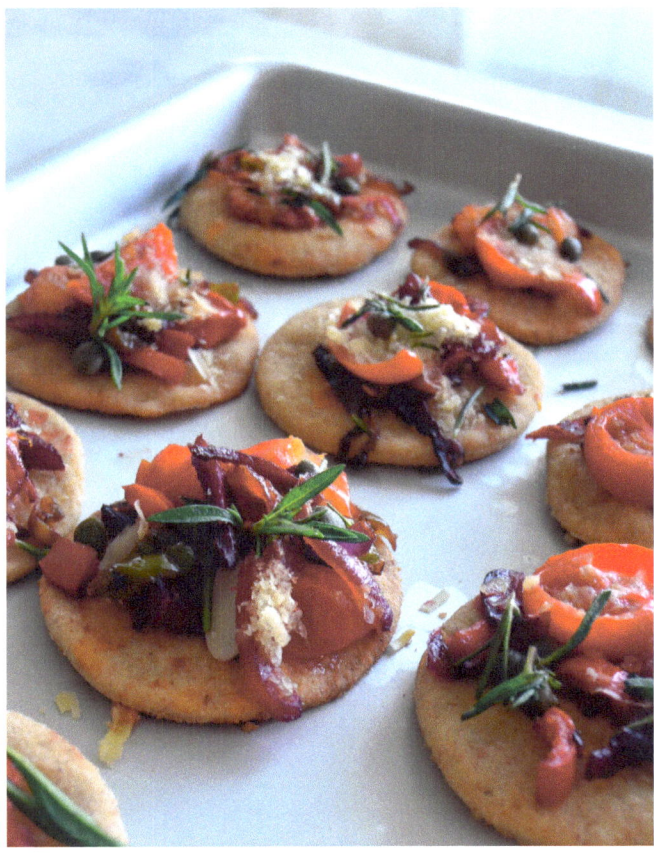
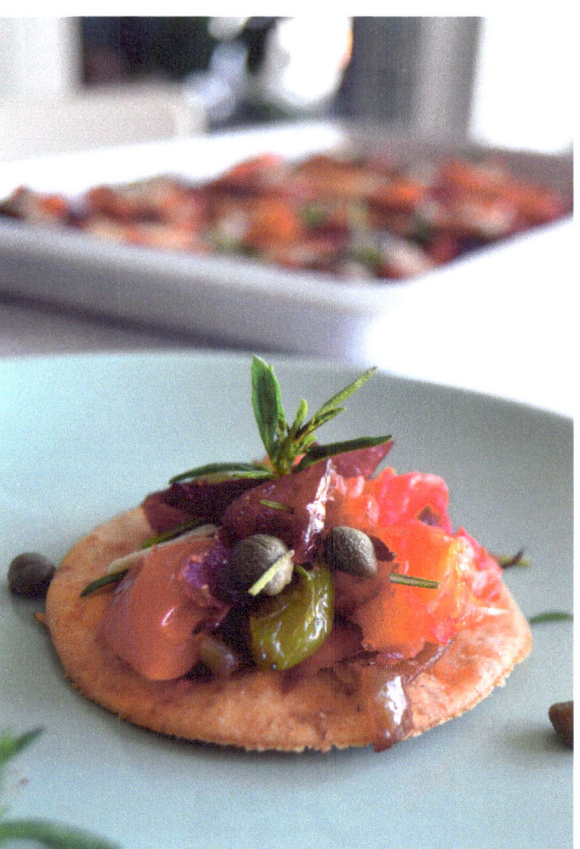

Ingredients

45 g fresh yeast
3 tbsp olive oil
2 tsp salt
1 cup warm water
3 cups whole wheat flour
1 tbsp coconut sugar

Toppings

1 medium red onion
1/2 cup cherry tomatoes
1 small beetroot
100 g shiitake mushrooms
1 large plum
1 large green california pepper
100 g vegan parmesan
30 g pine nuts
1-2 tbsp pickled capers
1 tbsp lemon juice
2 garlic cloves
1 tsp ground mustard
2 tbsp chopped fresh rosemary

1. Start dissolving the yeast in warm water, then add the olive oil, coconut sugar and salt. Mix together well. Then add the whole wheat flour, mix until get an elastic dough. Then knead well. Brush a bowl with olive oil. Place the dough in the bowl, cover with a warm towel, and let it triple in size in a warm place.
2. After one hour, transfer it to the refrigerator. Make your dough 4 days before you need it. The dough needs to be refrigerated for about 3 to 4 days before you start to work with it. It has a better flavor when it sets for a while or to use in the same day, knead dough with your hands for about 2-3 minutes. Divide 2 or 3 pieces. Roll them into a nice shape by using small round cutters. Bake in a skillet.
3. Heat up a large skillet pan, add olive oil, ground mustard, salt, lemon juice, thinly sliced red onions, mushrooms, plums, peppers, beets, pine nuts and garlic, cook over medium-high heat until golden brown. Top on your crust.
4. Spread shredded vegan cheese and cook for a minute or two. Decorate with fresh rosemary leaves and capers.

TIPS

Why does the local pizzeria's pizza taste better than the stuff you make at home? It's likely because their oven is hotter than yours. You should be baking your pizzas as hot as your oven will go- generally in the 230-260° C (450-500° F) range —but if you want to up your game even further, consider a higher heat approach like skillet-broiler method.

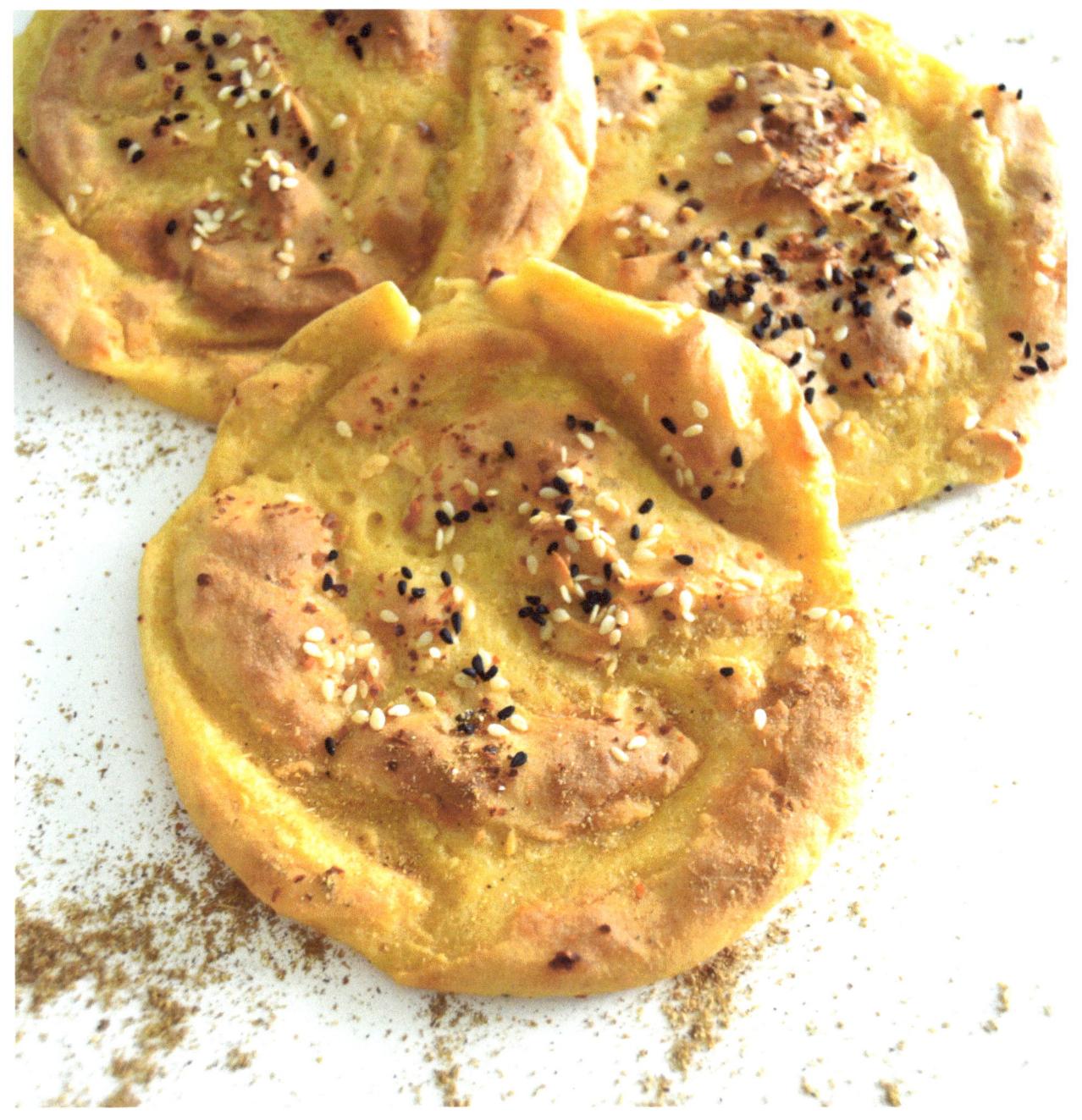

IRISH POTATOES

Cheesy and delicious these oven baked cheesy irish potatoes are quick, easy and are the absolute perfect side dish to any meal! You can make cheesy potatoes a number of ways by changing how you make them or what you use to make them.

Time - 1 hour
Serves - 4

375 g yukon gold potatoes
1 cup filtered water
1 tbsp maple or grape molasses
1/2 tsp onion powder
1/2 tsp ground coriander
1 tsp sea salt
1/2 tsp garlic powder
1 tbsp nutritional yeast
75 ml plant milk
4 tbsp rice flour (or tapioca)

Toppings
A pinch chili flakes
Black and white sesame seeds

1. Wash, peel and cut quarter potatoes.
2. Place in a deep pot, cover with water , bring to boil until soften.
3. Discard the rest of water. Let potatoes to cool for 10-15 min.
4. Place all ingredients into the food processor, mix on high speed until get smooth and sticky mixture.
6. Pre-heat oven to 180° C. Place parchment paper into the baking tray.
7. Scoop 2 tbsp dough pieces and place onto the parchment paper.
8. Top with chili flakes, black and white sesame.
9. Bake for 35-40 minutes or keep your eye out and remove from the oven once the tops are golden.
10. Cool for a few minutes before serving.

FIRST BITES

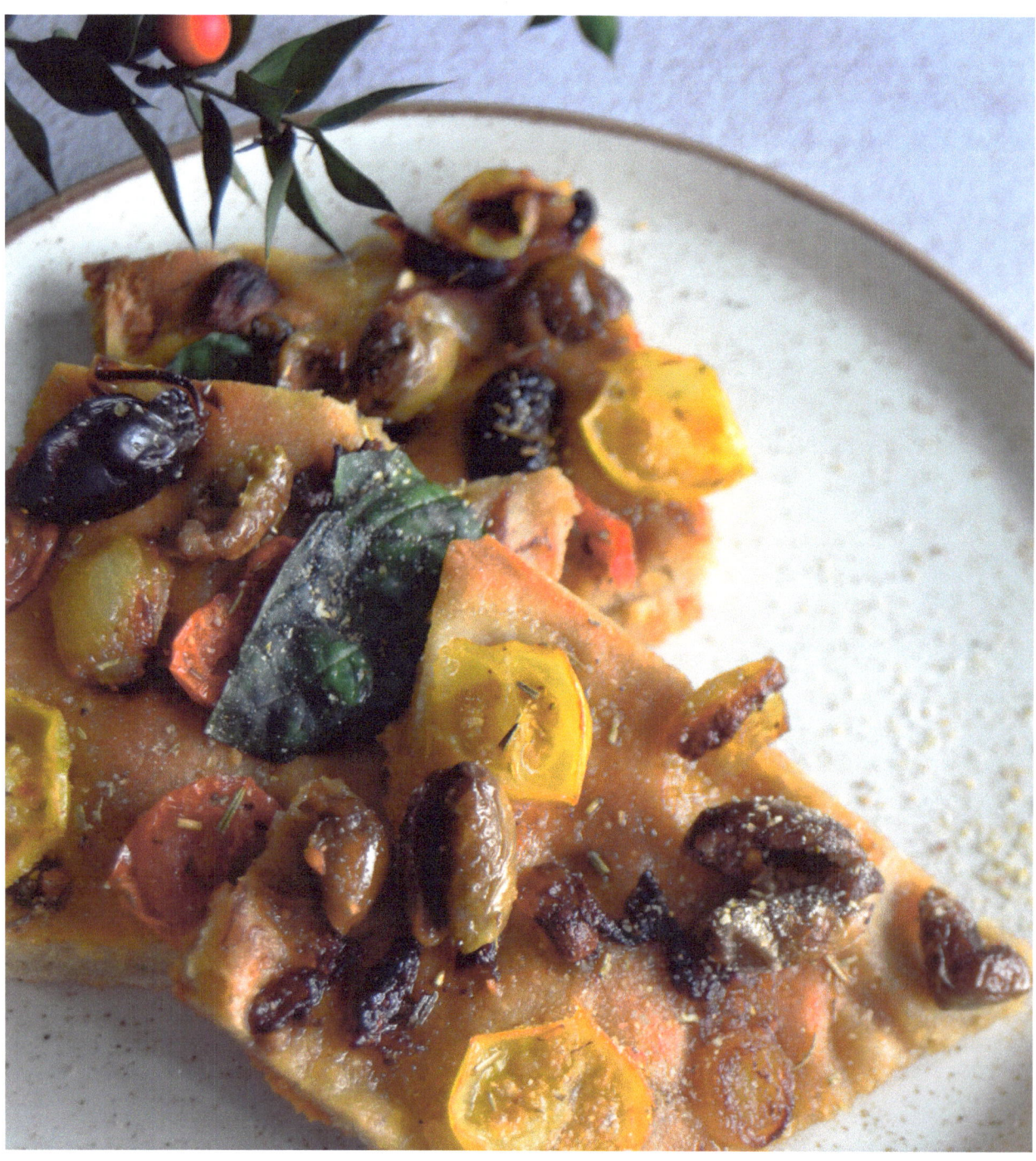

FOCACCIA BREAD

The secret to the best focaccia bread is great tasting olive oil. Since there is quite a bit used, the bread really takes on the flavor.

Time - 2 hour
Serves - 6-8 person

450 g whole wheat flour
10 g instant yeast
300 ml almond milk
1 tsp sea salt
1 cup cherry tomatoes
1/2 cup olives
1/2 cup olive oil
2 tsp rosemary chopped
6-7 shallot chopped
2 tsp garlic powder

1. In a large bowl, whisk together yeast, almond milk and 1 tbsp olive oil.
2. Pour flour in to the bowl. Mix together. Stir well with a wooden spoon. Cover bowl with a plastic wrap, let it rest for 30-35 minutes or until it begins to get bubbly.
3. Knead dough with your hands, turn out on to a work surface. Knead well again. Place it into bowl , cover and let to rest it again for 10-15 minutes. Preheat oven to 50° C. Place bowl in to the oven for 40 minutes or until it has doubled in size.
4. Remove bowl from the oven. Transfer it to a work surface. Knead and strech out with your hands. When the dough is smooth, coat it in a thin layer of 1 tbsp olive oil. Preheat oven to 220° C. Put a parchment paper in a pan. Flatten and shape the dough in a baking pan. Strech it into the corners.
5. Make deep holes with a teaspoon to put olives and tomatoes. Cut olives and tomatoes in two. Push them into the holes.
6. Drizzle a little bit extra olive oil if desired. Sprinkle sea salt and rosemary.
7. Bake for 18-20 minutes or until golden browned. Remove from the oven, let it cool before serving.
8. Enjoy alone or serve with nut cheeses.

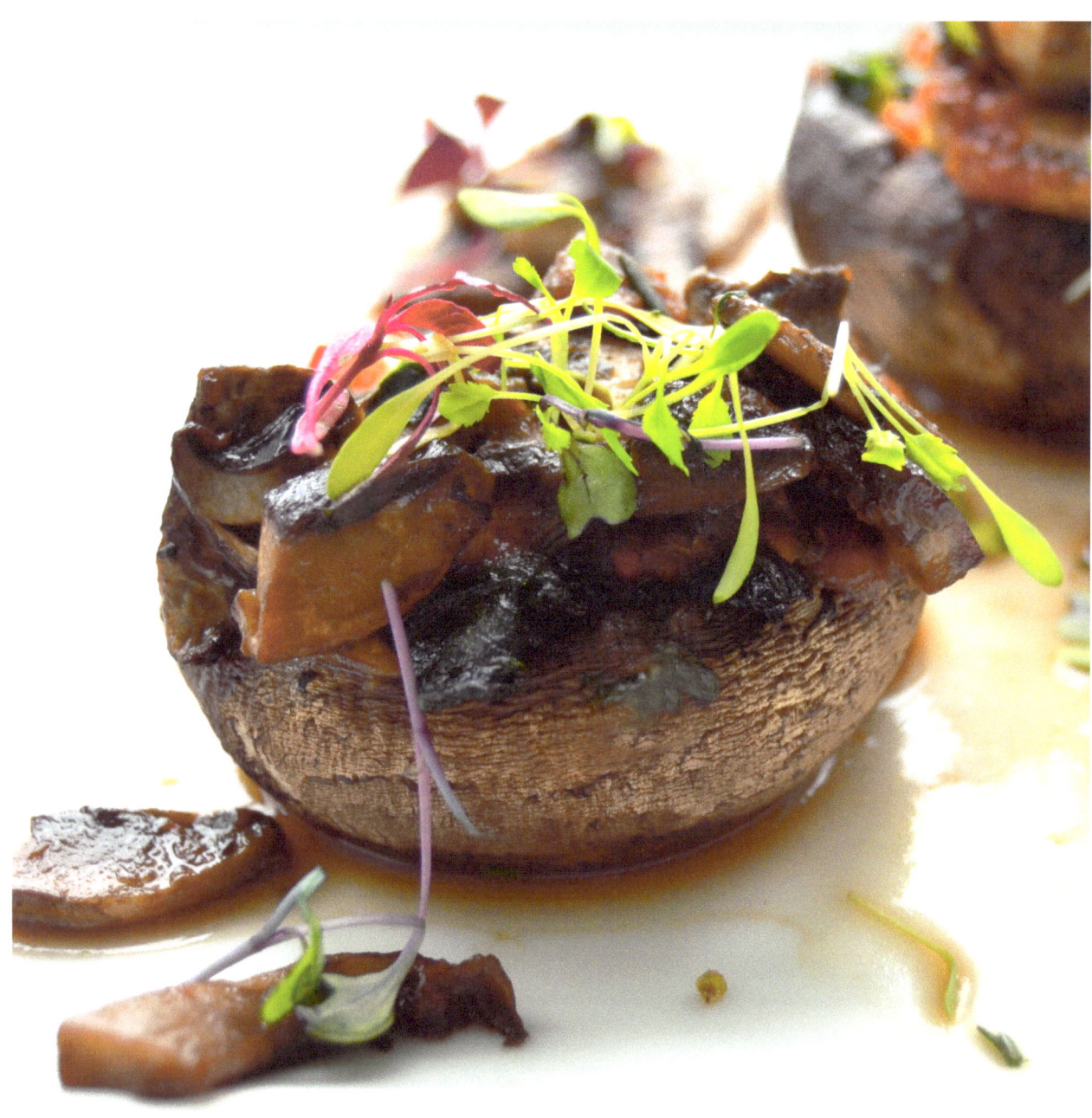

PORTOBELLO MUSHROOMS

Portobello mushrooms have a robust meaty texture making them good for roasting, baking and stuffing.

Time - 1 hour
Serves - 3 as a side

Ingredients
7 large portabello mushrooms
200 g fresh spinach
2 tbsp olive oil
1 medium onion
2 tbsp soy sauce or tamari
60 g vegan parmesan
2 red bell pepper
Microgreens to serve
1 tsp salt

1. Brush and clean your mushrooms, set aside one cap to saute , spray remaining 6 caps with olive oil cooking spray on both sides.
2. Preheat oven to 200° C.
3. Wash your veggies and drain. Chop onion or leek, cut the cap you set aside before , into small pieces. Chop red pepper.
4. Shred vegan parmesan very thinly. Place in medium bowl, set aside.
5. Line a parchment paper in a baking tray. Place mushrooms onto the pan. Bake for 15 minutes or until turn golden brown. In a large pan, saute leek and peppers together in olive oil.
6. Add chopped mushrooms, soy sauce and spinach. Cook on medium heat for about 4-5 minutes. Add salt and black pepper, stir and remove from the oven.
7. Using a small spoon, fill your mushrooms with spinach mixture. Spread shredded vegan parmesan over the mushrooms.
8. Bake for 10 minutes in the oven. Decorate with microgreens, serve!

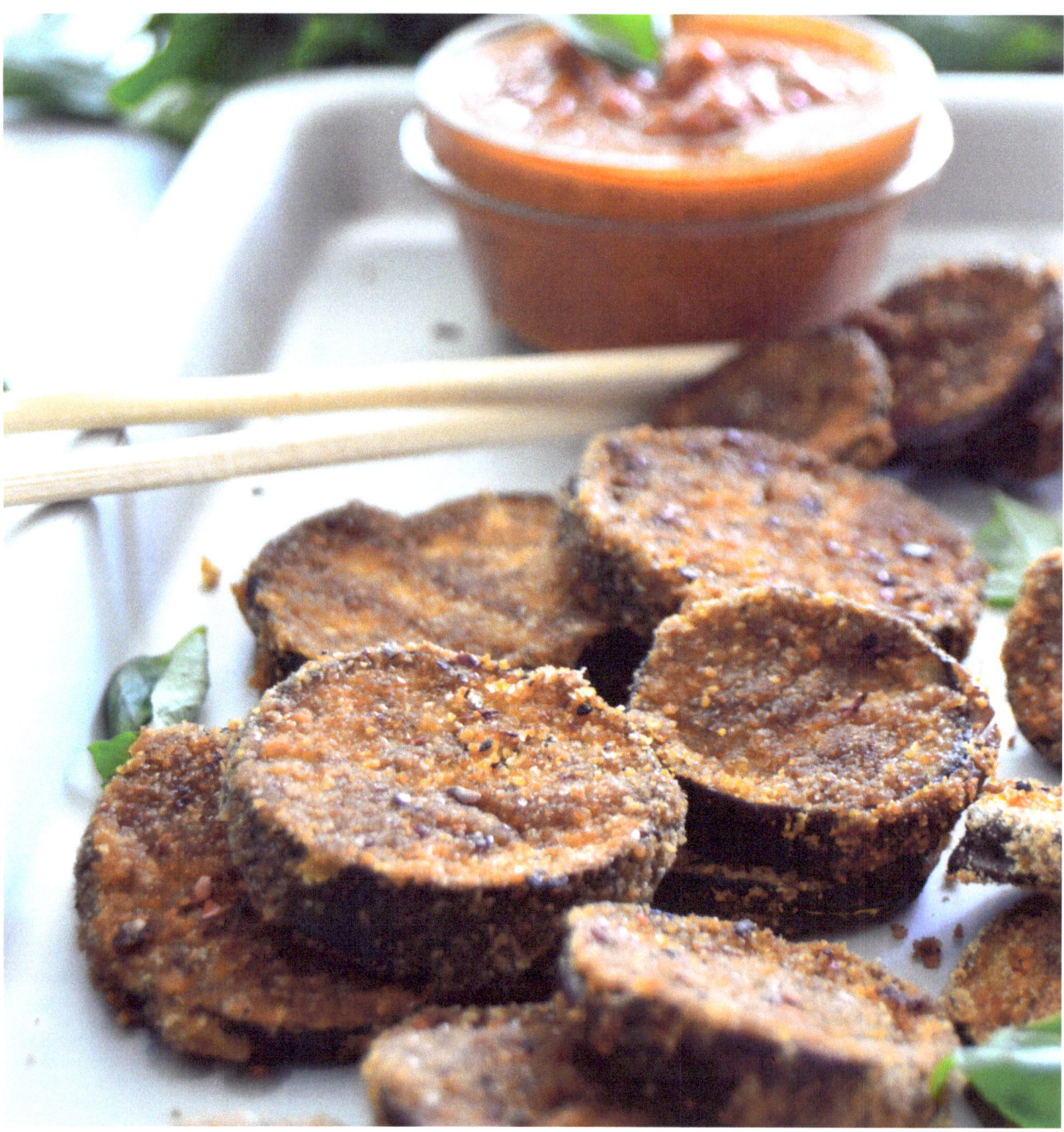

CHRUNCY EGGPLANTS

Time - 20 min prep + 50 min baking
Serves - 2-3

Ingredients
3 medium eggplants
1 cup bread crumbs
2 tbsp ground flaxseed
5 tbsp water
1 tsp sea salt
1 tbsp olive oil
1/4 tsp blackpepper
1 tsp red pepper flakes

Sauce
1 small onion chopped
2 large tomatoes
1 tbsp tomato paste
1 tsp garlic powder
1 tsp oregano
1 tsp chili
1 tsp salt
2 tbsp olive oil
1 medium carrot chopped
6-7 kalamata olives
1/4 bunch fresh basil chopped
1/8 tsp blackpepper

1. Pre-heat oven to 200° C.
2. Cut the eggplants 3/8" thick.
3. Place them in a bowl, cover with water and let them rest for about 1 hours in order to remove their bitterness.
4. Then strain and dry your eggplant slices. Place them in a bowl.
5. In a small bowl, mix ground flaxseed and water. Let it rest in the fridge for 10 minutes.
6. In a medium bowl place the breadcrumbs.
7. Dip the sliced eggplants in the flax seed liquid first. Then dip it in the breadcrumb to coat.
8. Then place the coated eggplants on the baking sheet again. Drizzle with olive oil. Sprinkle some salt and peppers. Repeat process for all.
9. Bake your eggplants in the oven for 30 minutes then flip up and continute to bake for 20 minutes or until golden.
10. Place all sauce ingredients into the food processor, mix on high speed until everything combined well.
11. Pour mixture into the sauce pan, cook on medium heat for 3-4 minutes. Place it into a small sauce bowl. Serve with your baked eggplants.

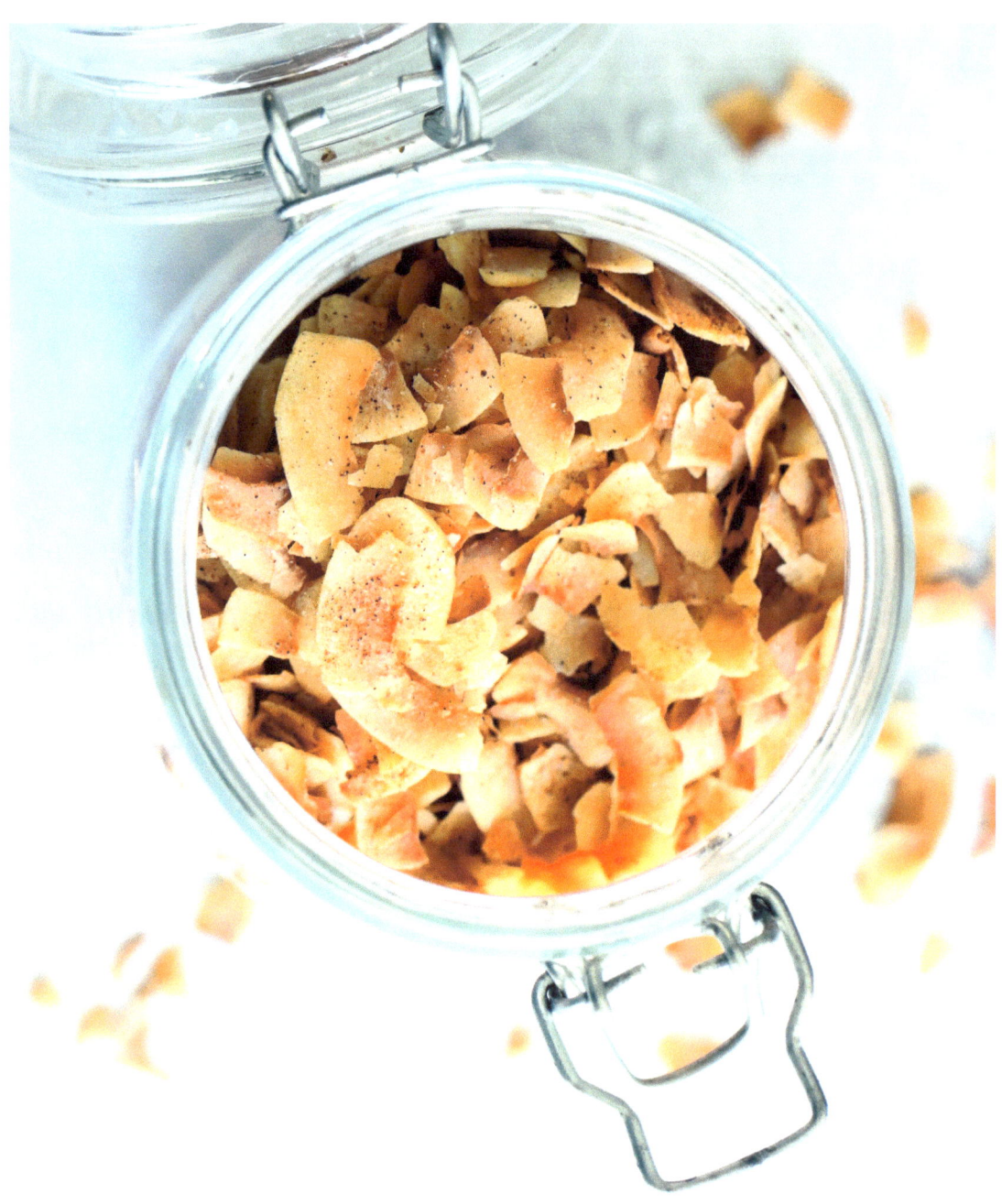

SPICY COCONUT BACON

Time - 45 minutes
Serves - 4-6

Ingredients
200 g fresh coconut meat
1/2 tsp ground coriander
1/4 tsp dried tarragon
1 tbsp nutritional yeast
1 tbsp apple cider vinegar
1 tbsp tamari
1 tsp smoked paprika
1/2 tsp chili
1/2 tsp salt

1. Pre-heat oven to 175° C.
2. Place a parchment paper onto the baking pan.
3. To crack the coconut, wrap the coconut in a towel and hold it. Turn the coconut and tap it with a mallet until it cracks. Split the coconut shell and place it cut side down. Hit the coconut with the mallet to loosen the meat. Run a knife between the shell and the meat to free it.
4. Then using a mandolin slicer, thinly slice the coconut meat.
5. In a large bowl, mix all ingredients well. Add coconut meats into the bowl, toss together with the herbs.
6. Place coconut shavings onto the parchment paper, bake for 10 minutes or until flakes are golden brown.
7. Then flip them and cook for about 10-12 minutes. If you need crispy, then cook for 15 minutes.
8. Let it cool and serve them with stir-fry veggies, salads or enjoy as a snack.

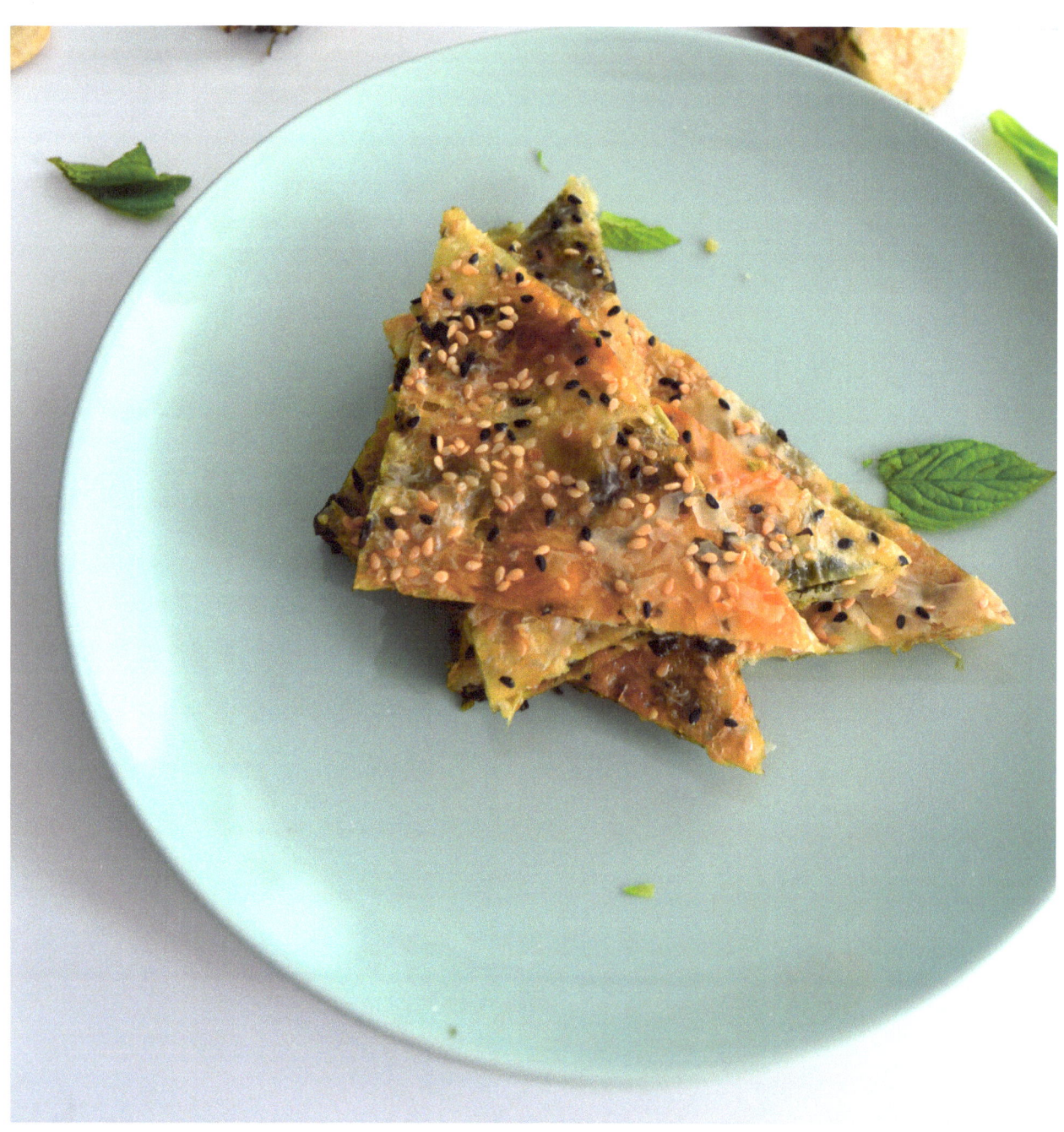

PHYLLO BÖREK WITH SPINACH

Phyllo (also spelled filo), which means "leaf" in Greek, is tissue-thin sheets of dough that have very little fat. Many popular Turkish and Greek dishes, such as baklava and spanakopita, are made with phyllo dough. The sheets are usually brushed with oil and then layered together. When it bakes up, the layers get airy, crisp, and flaky. The main thing to know about working with phyllo dough is to keep it from drying out. Keep the sheets covered with a towel while you're working!

Time - 1 hour
Serves - 4-6

Ingredients
400 g spinach
1 medium onion finely chopped
3 garlic cloves minced
1 small carrot finely chopped
2 medium red bell pepper chopped
8-10 thin sheets of phyllo
1 cup almond milk
2 tbsp soy sauce
4 tbsp olive oil

1. Lightly fry onions , red bell peppers, carrot and garlic cloves in a little oil. Fry on medium heat for 4-5 minutes until caramelized then add the spinach. Cook until excess water has evaporated. Set aside.
2. In a medium bowl, stir together almond milk and 1 tbsp oil.
3. Place a pyhllo on the bottom of the baking pan. Spread almond milk oil mixture until completely wet. Lightly brush sheet with the spinach mixture using a small pastry brush. Lay another sheet of phyllo dough on top, brush with almond milk mixture.
4. Add one more layer and repeat process for the remaining 5 sheets too. Brush almond milk oil mixture on top floor until fully wet. Spread black and white sesame seeds.
5. Bake in pre-heat oven to 220° C for 30 minutes or till golden brown. Cut in triangles and serve warm!

To freeze: prepare, fill the pastry. Do not coat with liquid wash or bake. Place the unbaked pastries in a pyrex separating each layer of pastry with a piece of parchment paper to keep them from freezing together. Freeze. When ready to bake, take the pastry out of the freezer and arrange them on a baking sheet sprayed with nonstick oil. Coat with thin layer of plant based milk wash and sesame or poppy seeds, if desired. Bake at 220° C for 20-30 minutes till golden brown.

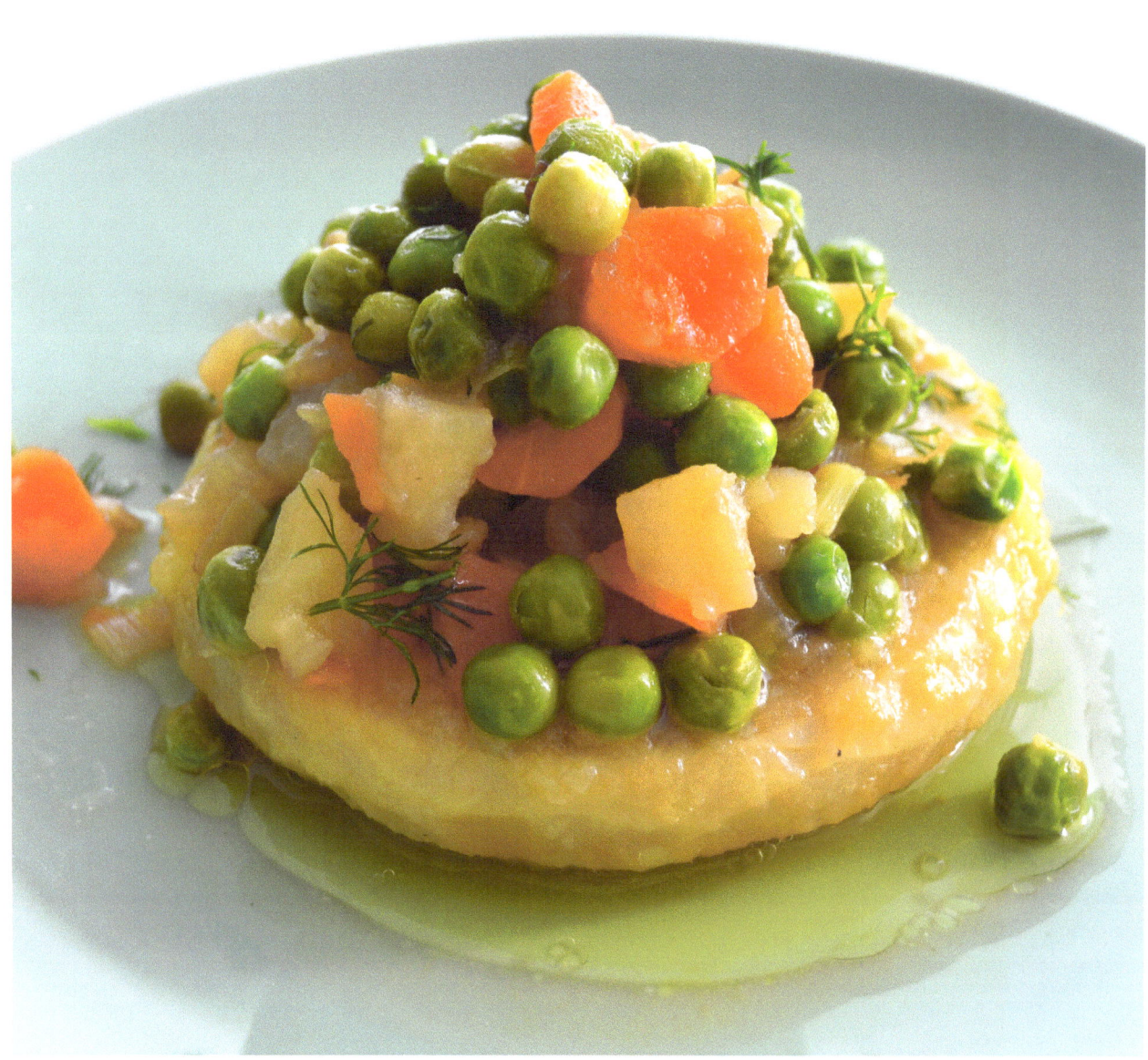

ARTICKHOKE WITH PEAS

This artichoke pea dish is a spring-summer starter dish that is very popular in Aegean region of Turkey and in Greece. So easy to make and satisfying!

Time - 30 minutes
Serves - 4

Ingredients
4 pieces artichoke bottoms peeled
1 tbsp olive oil
1 carrot cubes
1 cup fresh or frozen green peas
2 slices of fresh pineapples
1/2 tsp salt
1 tbsp lemon juice
2 tbsp pineapple juice
1 tbsp coconut sugar
4 tbsp warm water
Fresh dill to serve

1. Cut carrots and pineapples into small cubes. Place on a non-stick pan. Then add the peas and little olive oil. Cook for 2-3 minutes contantly stirring. Once lightly caramelized, add some water.
2. Cook for 5-6 minutes or until soften enough and carrots and pineapples absorb the water content.
3. Mix coconut sugar, pineapple juice and lemon juice in a clean pot. Cook until caramelized and soften enough.
4. Place peeled artichoke bottoms in a deep pot. Cover with water, cook for 10 minutes or until tender. Once cooked, remove from the pot.
5. Add the carrot, pineapple and peas on the top of artichokes.
6. Pour the sauce over the artichokes. Sprinkle some fresh dill. Serve warm or cold. Add some extra olive oil if desired.

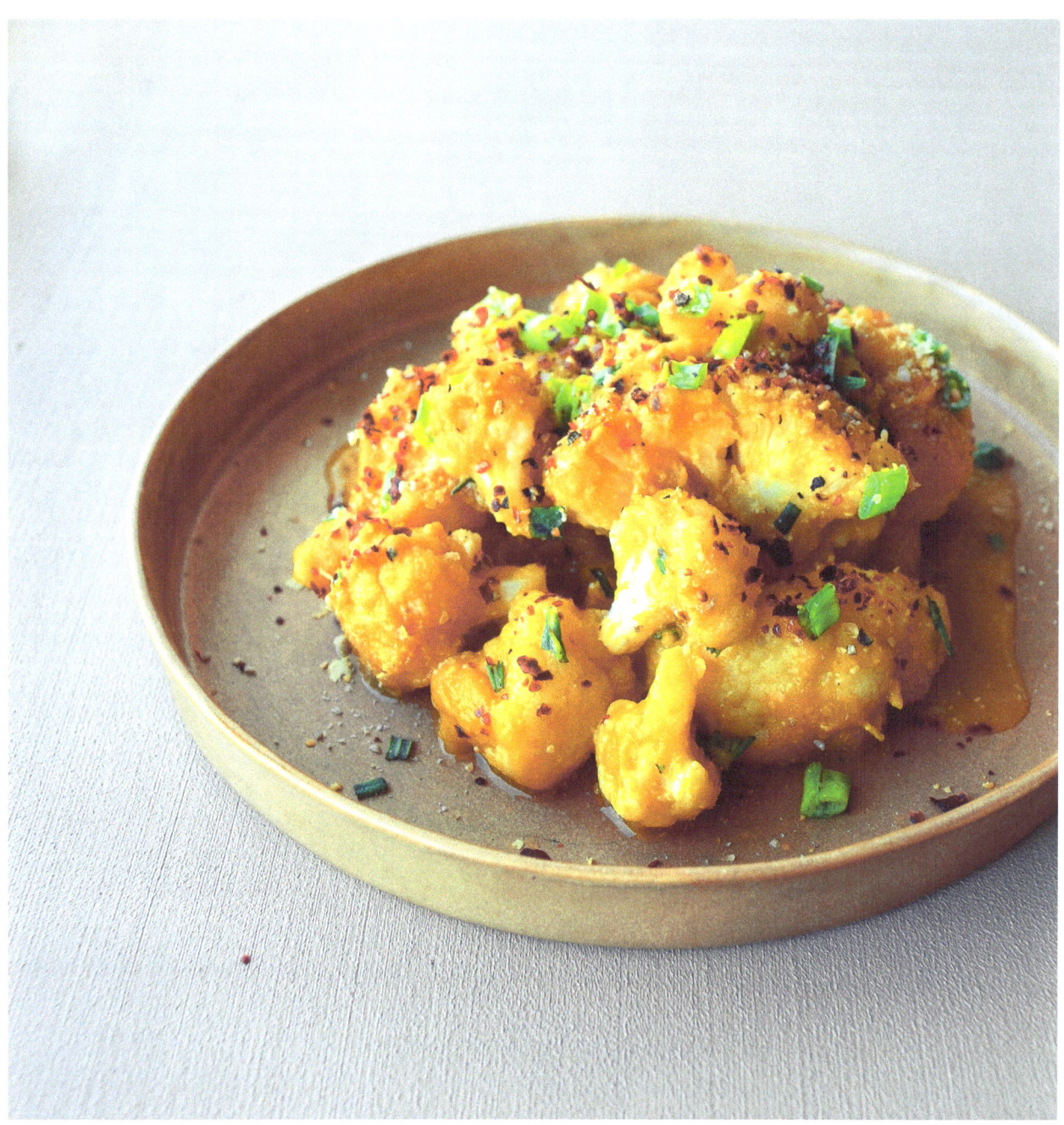

CAULIFLOWER WITH PUMPKIN SAUCE

Time - 10 min prep + 25 min baking
Serves - 2 person

1/2 head of cauliflower
1/2 tsp red pepper flakes
2 tsp garlic powder
A generous amount of salt and black pepper to taste
Green onions chopped to serve
2 tbsp freshly chopped rosemary
1/4 cup hopped walnuts or vegan parmesan

Pumpkin Sauce
500 g pumpkin
1 cup almond milk
3 garlic cloves minced
1 red onion chopped
1 bay leaf
1/2 cup vegetable broth
1 tsp salt
1 tsp whole blackpepper

1. Cut the head of cauliflower into small florets. Wash and drain. Set aside.
2. In a pot, add 2-3 tbsp vegetable broth or olive oil , then saute the onions and garlic until soften.
3. Cut your pumpkin into small pieces. Then add to the pot.
4. Pour the vegetable broth over the pumpkins. Add the bay leaf and black pepper seeds. Bring to boil until pumpkins are soften.
5. Once cooked, transfer to a high speed blender, add the almond milk and blend until smooth puree.
6. Place your cauliflower florets in a casserole tray. Top with pumpkin sauce.
7. Bake the casserole for 15-20 minutes, until the sauce becomes thick enough.
8. Once cooked, remove from the oven. Sprinkle some chopped nuts or vegan parmesan, green onions, rosemary. Adjust the salt and pepper. Serve immediately!

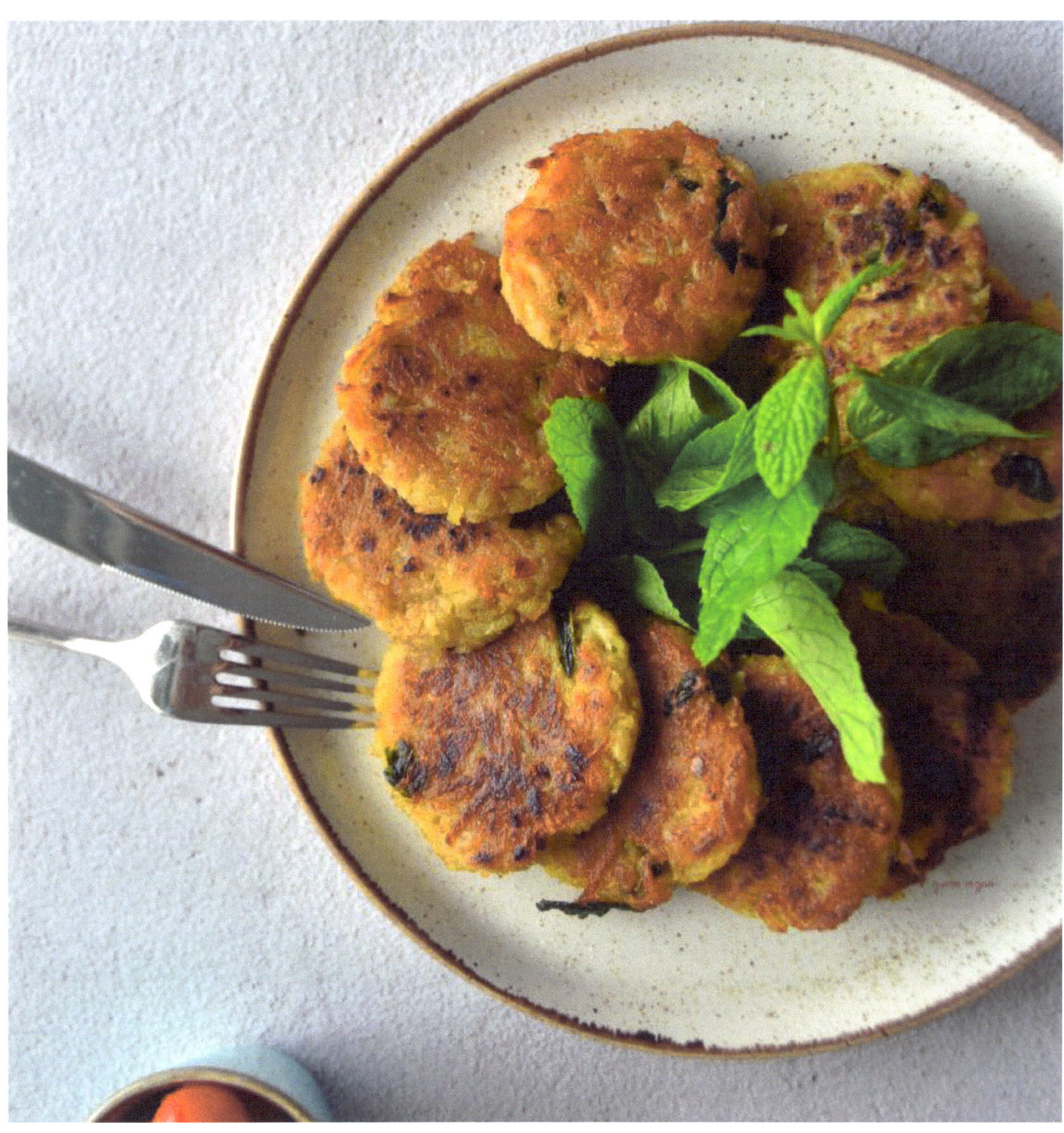

CELERIAC HASHBROWNS

Time - 10 min prep + 25 min baking
Serves - 2-3

Hashbrowns
1 large celeriac
1 large yukon gold potato
1/2 tsp salt
5-6 leaves fresh basil
1/4 tsp baking soda
4 tbsp whole-wheat flour or use gluten-free flour mixture
2 tsp lupin powder or ground flaxseed
6 tbsp water
Olive oil to fry

Chili Sauce
1 cup tomato sauce
1 tablespoon coconut sugar
1/4 teaspoon garlic powder
2 tablespoons distilled white vinegar
1/2 teaspoon chili powder
1/4 teaspoon onion powder

1. Wash the celery roots and potato. Grate them in a large mixing bowl.
2. Wash, drain and cut basil leaves into small pieces.
3. In a small bowl, mix lupin powder and water together.
4. Add chili pepper, basil leaves, baking soda, whole wheat flour, lupin mixture and salt into the bowl. Toss with grated celery potato mixture. Knead with your hands well.
5. Pour the olive oil into the frying pan until the bottom of the pan is just coated in oil. Heat the pan over medium-high heat and add 1 tablespoon of the hashbrown mixture, flattening it and evenly spreading it out over the surface of the pan with a spatula.
6. Fry for 5-6 minutes on each side, until golden brown. When they are fried, remove the hashbrown patties from the pan and place it on a plate lined with paper towels.
7. To make chili sauce, whisk tomato sauce, brown sugar, vinegar, chili powder, garlic powder, and onion powder together in a bowl.
8. Serve your hashbrownes with chili sauce or plant-based yogurt.

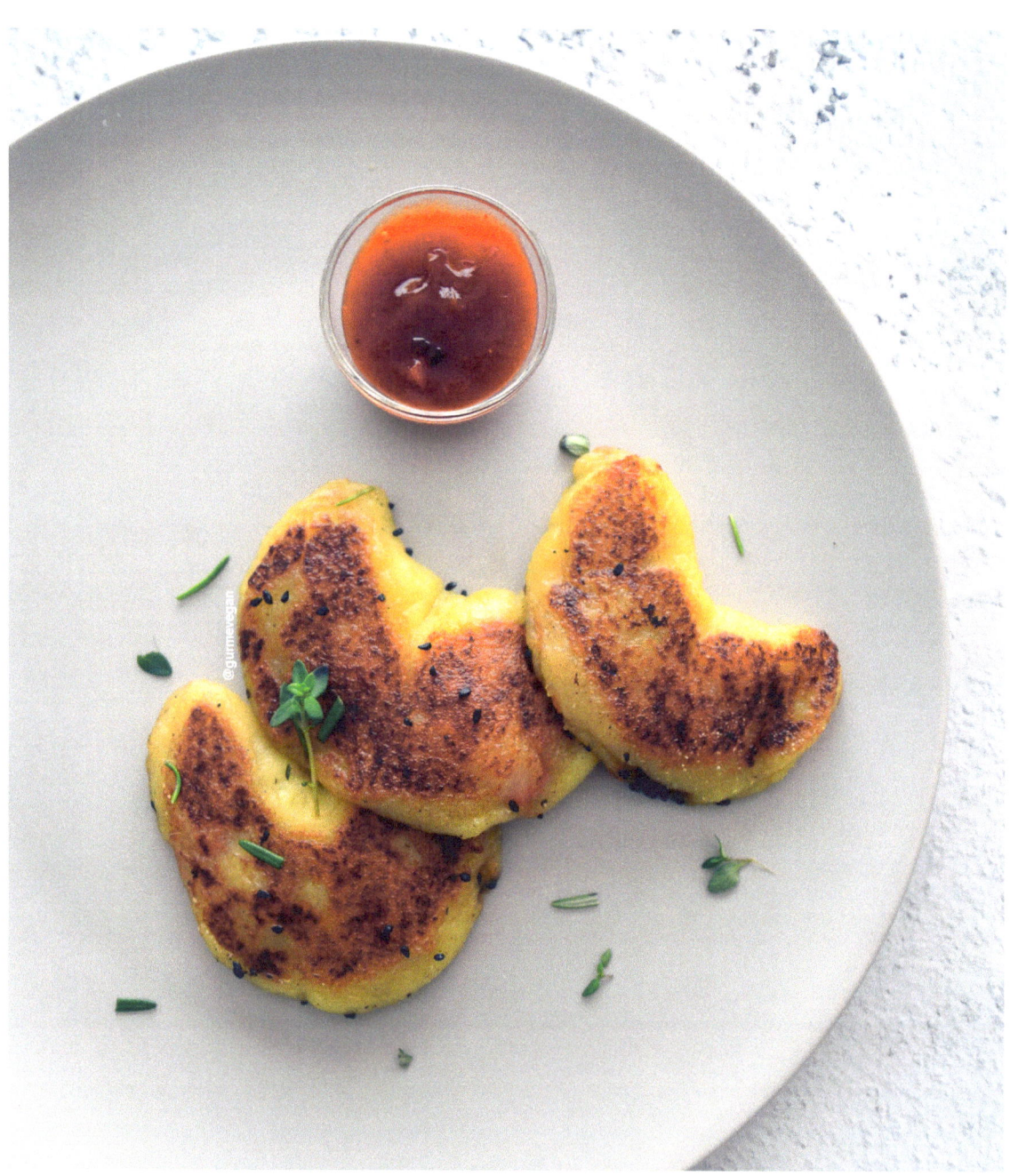

POTATO POCKETS

Time - 40 minutes
Serves - 2-3

Ingredients
3 large potatoes (approx. 700 g)
3 tbsp of tapioca
15 g psyllium powder
1 tbsp olive oil
1 tsp of himalayan salt

Filling
1 tbsp olive oil
1 medium red onion
1 medium carrot
3 cloves of garlic
2 tbsp capers
2 sprigs of fresh rosemary
2 medium tomatoes

1. Boil the potatoes until soft, then peel, cut into small pieces and transfer to the food processor. Add tapioca, salt, psyllium powder and olive oil and mix well at high speed. Remove the dough from the food processor and divide it into small balls and set aside.
2. Cut the onions, carrots and garlic and transfer into the pan. Saute with a tablespoon of olive oil. When softened, add the tomatoes cut into cubes and cook a little more. Add the latest capers and freshly chopped rosemary and stir, remove from heat.
3. Roll small balls using a rolling pin. Place a tablespoon filling. Close the ends and make a moon shape. Repeat the process for the rest of the dough.
4. Fry each side in a pan with a little olive oil. Serve with BBQ if desired.

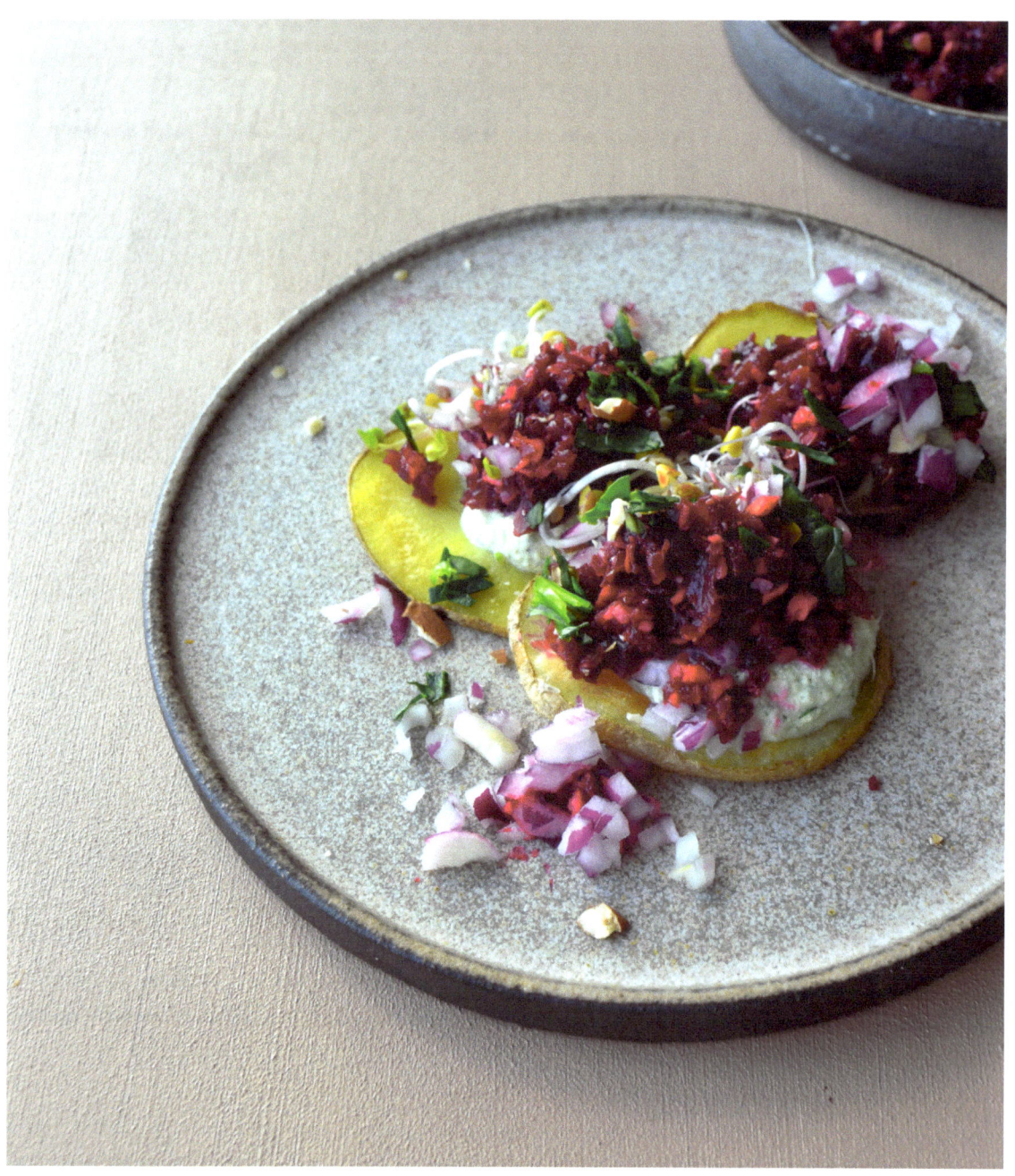

POTATOES WITH BEETROOT PESTO AND HEMP CREAM

Time - 50 minutes
Serves - 3-4

Ingredients
500 g potatoes
1 tsp baking soda (it is cruical ingredient to make potatoes crispy)
2 tsp salt
1 tsp onion powder
1 tsp garlic powder
1 tsp dried rosemary
Chopped red onion to serve

Beet Pesto
2 beetroots
1/2 bunch fresh parsley
Juice of whole lemon
Salt and pepper to taste
1/4 cup crushed walnuts

Hemp Cream
1 cup hemp hearts
1 tbsp dijon mustard
Juice of whole lemon
Salt and pepper to taste
Water to thin

1. Wash your potatoes and cut into small pieces. Preheat oven to 200° C.
2. Place the potatoes in a pot, cover with water. Add 1 tsp baking soda and 1 tsp salt. Bring to boil for about 10 minutes.
3. Then strain the water. Add 1 tsp salt, onion, garlic and dried rosemary. Give it a good toss.
4. Transfer the potatoes onto a baking tray lined parchment paper.
5. Bake in the oven for 25-30 minutes or until crispy enough and golden.
6. Place all beet pesto ingredients in a food processor, process until rice-like texture.
7. Place all hemp cream ingredients in a blender, blend until creamy.
8. Serve with your potatoes with beet pesto, hemp cream and chopped red onion

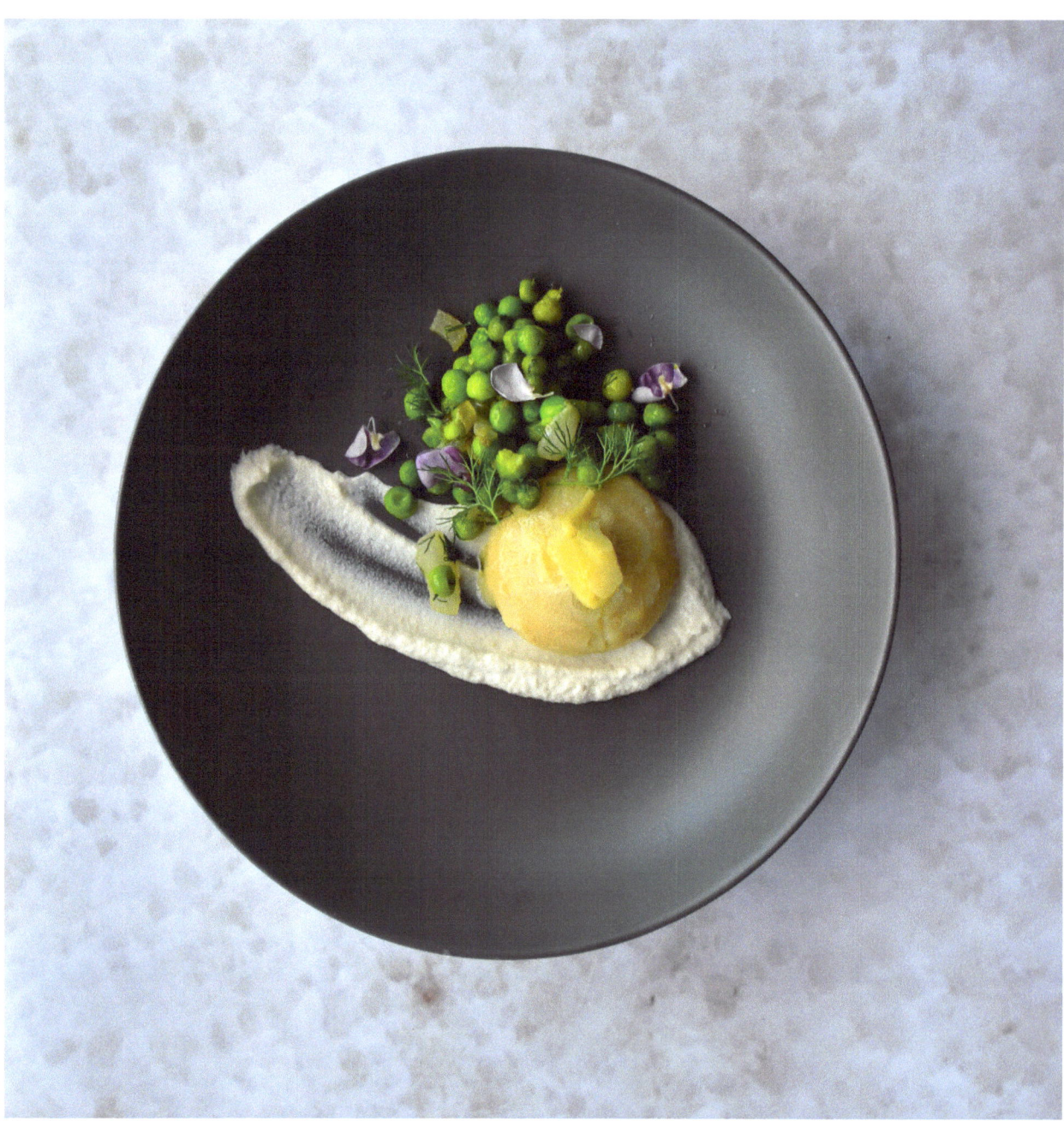

ARTICHOKE WITH PEAS

Ingredients
10 medium sized artichokes
1 kg peas
500 g spring onions
4-5 tbsp extra virgin olive oil
2 bunches of parsley or dill
juice from 2 small lemons

1. Clean the artichokes as follows: remove the stalks and the hard leaves from the artichokes. Cut the hard edges of the leaves, remove the fuzzy choke, cut them and put them in a bowl of water and juice of one lemon so as not to blacken.

2. Chop the onion and dill.

3. Heat someolive oil. Reduce heat and add the onion until golden. Add the peas and the artichoke hearts and sauté for 5 minutes.

4. Add the rest of the ingredients except for the lemon juice. 5. Add water, as much as is needed in order to cover half of the ingredient. Close the lid and allow to simmer until the vegetables soften – for about 45 minutes.

5. Finally, add the lemon juice, salt and pepper. Serve with vegan yogurt or sunflower seed cream if desired.

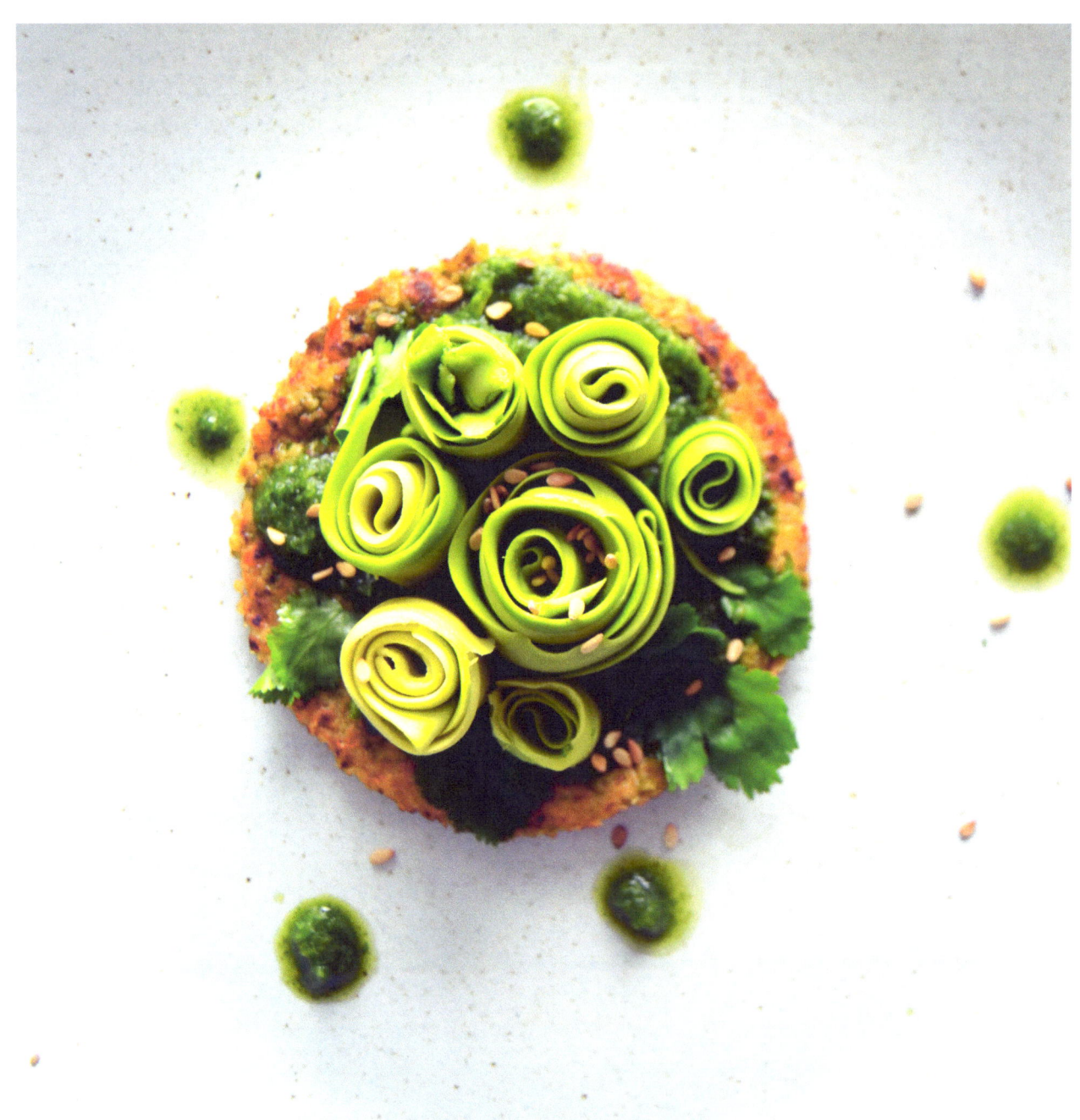

MOONG DAL CHILLA

Just like Dosa in South India, Chilla is an absolute favourite Breakfast recipe in North India. Almost every North Indian household makes Chilla for breakfast with a hot cup of tea or coffee or sometimes even for lunch during weekdays, as it is extremely easy to make and nutritious too.

Time - 40 minutes
Serves - 3-4

Ingredients
1 cup mung lentils soaked overnight
1 small onion
4-5 cherry tomatoes
1 tsp garlic puree
1 medium red bell pepper
1 tsp ginger puree
1/4 tsp turmeric
1/2 tsp salt
2 tbsp olive oil
1/2 avocado
Sesame and coriander leaves to decorate

Green Chutney
1 cup chopped coriander leaves
1 green chili
1/ 2 tsp ginger puree
1/2 lemon juice
1/4 teaspoon salt

1. Place the mung lentils into the water overnight and soak at least 6 hours. Then rinse and drain them.
2. Place mung lentils into the food processor, add all remaining ingredients (except avocado, sesame and coriander) and blend on high speed until you get smooth mixture.
3. Once the mixture is smooth, heat and spread some olive oil on the pan.
4. Pour it on the pan evenly.
5. Cook on slow to medium heat for about a minute. Then flip the side and cook for another minute until crispy.
6. Repeat the process for to make more chillas.
7. Place all chutney ingredients into the food processor mix on high speed until puree. Then pour mixture over the crepes.
8. Peel a slightly ripe avocado (shouldn't be soft) using a standart peeler. Roll them with your hands and give a rose shape. Top on the chutney.
9. Sprinkle some sesame and mint or coriander leaves , serve!

GOURMET VEGAN

SOUPS

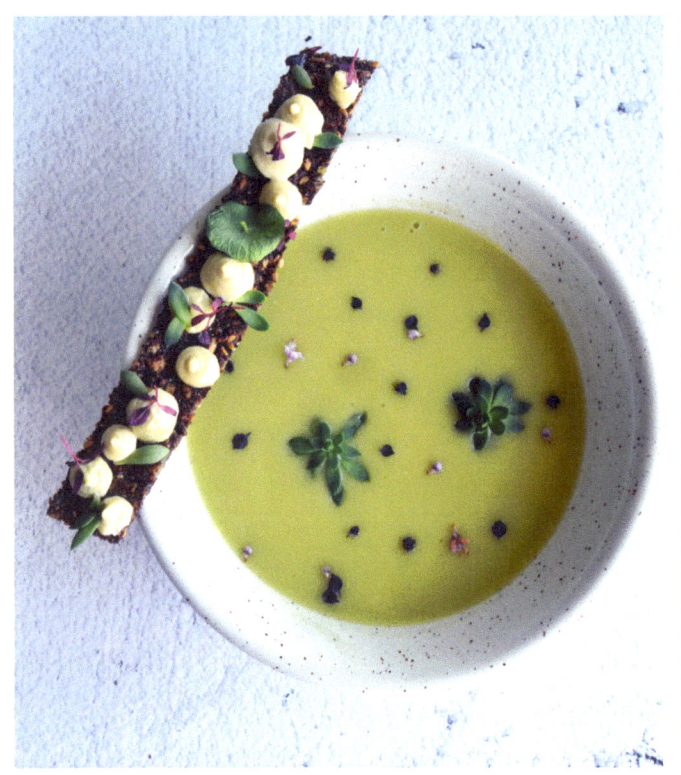
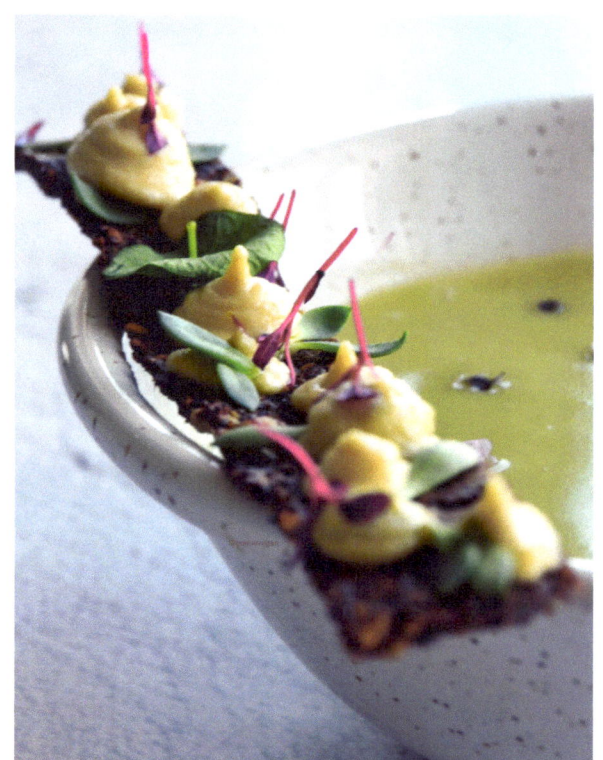

BROAD BEAN SOUP

Time - 50 minutes
Serves - 2-3

Ingredients
350 g broad beans
1 large head artichoke
1 large red onion
2 large garlic cloves
1 large carrot
2 tbsp olive oil
750 ml vegetable stock or water
Salt & pepper to taste
1/2 lemon juice
Gangnam tops for garnish
Nasturtium leaves for garnish
Amaranth microgreens for garnish

1. Clean and cut your onion, garlic and carrots. Place in a large pot. Cook with a little olive oil until get browned.
2. Clean the artichoke till you reach the heart. Then cut in half vertical, clean fuzzy center with a teaspoon and remove. (Keep them in lemon water until use to avoid getting darken)
3. Transfer artichoke heart to the pot over the browned carrots, pour the vegetable stock. Bring it to boil then simmer for 30-35 minutes.
4. Let it cool down for 20 minutes.
6. Peel the skin of the broad beans one by one. (can be done overnight)
7. Add the broad beans to a clean pot and cook with a little bit water until soft. Be careful not to overcook them. Otherwise, they lose the bright green color. We want them bright and vibrant.
9. Once done, blend the cooked broad beans and artichoke carrot mixture together until smooth. Using a strainer, strain the soup if desired. Adjust seasoning.
10. Add some lemon juice for a tangy flavour. Cook for 2-3 minutes. Divide between bowls. Decorate with edible flowers if desired.
11. Serve with seed cracker and garlic confit. (see the recipe on the next page)

Crackers

45 g flax seeds freshly grounded
15 g white sesame seeds
10 g poppy seeds
15 g chia seeds
15 g sunflower seeds
1 tbsp psyllium husk powder
Salt and pepper to taste
120 ml warm water

Instructions

1. Mix all ingredients in a large bowl and add 120 ml warm water and mix well. Then let it rest for 15 minutes until absorbs all water.
2. Place the dough in between two baking paper and roll it evenly. It should be around 5-6 mm thick. Avoid making it too thin otherwise they crack during baking.
3. Remove the baking paper on top but keep the one underneath. Cut into long pieces.
4. Bake at 175° C for about 8-10 minutes or until completely dry and crispy.

Garlic Confit

70 g garlic peeled
100 ml olive oil
2 spring onion chives
1 spring thyme

Instructions

1. Place all ingredients in a sauce pot. Bring it to simmer but not boil.
2. Simmer at the lowest heat possible for about and hour. Garlic should be very soft but not caramelized.
3. Let it cool down. Strain the confit garlic but keep the oil.
4. Mash garlic, then transfer into a pipping bag.
5. Decorate your crackers with garlic drops. Garnish with amarant microgreens, nasturtium and gangnam tops or other preferred edible flowers and herbs if desired.

ASPARAGUS SOUP

Time - 30 minutes
Serves - 3-4

Ingredients
1 tbsp oil
1 shallot, diced
1 clove of garlic, minced
1 tsp green curry paste
500 g green asparagus
1 cup coconut milk
1/2 cup water
1/2 tsp salt
1/8 tsp ground pepper
1 tsp nutritional yeast

1. Heat the oil in a large skillet over medium heat.
2. Once hot, add the shallot, garlic, and green curry paste. Cook for 3-5 minutes, or until shallots are soft and golden brown.
3. In the meantime, dice the asparagus into 1-inch pieces and rinse them under cold water. Add to the skillet and cook for 5 minutes, stirring regularly to prevent sticking.
4. Pour in the coconut milk, water, salt, and ground pepper.
5. Cover and let simmer over medium heat fo 7-8 minutes, or until the asparagus are soft.
6. Transfer to a blender, add the nutritional yeast and blend on high speed until smooth and creamy. Taste and adjust salt if needed. Serve hot topped with toasted pine nuts, some quinoa, and optionally some sautéed asparagus.

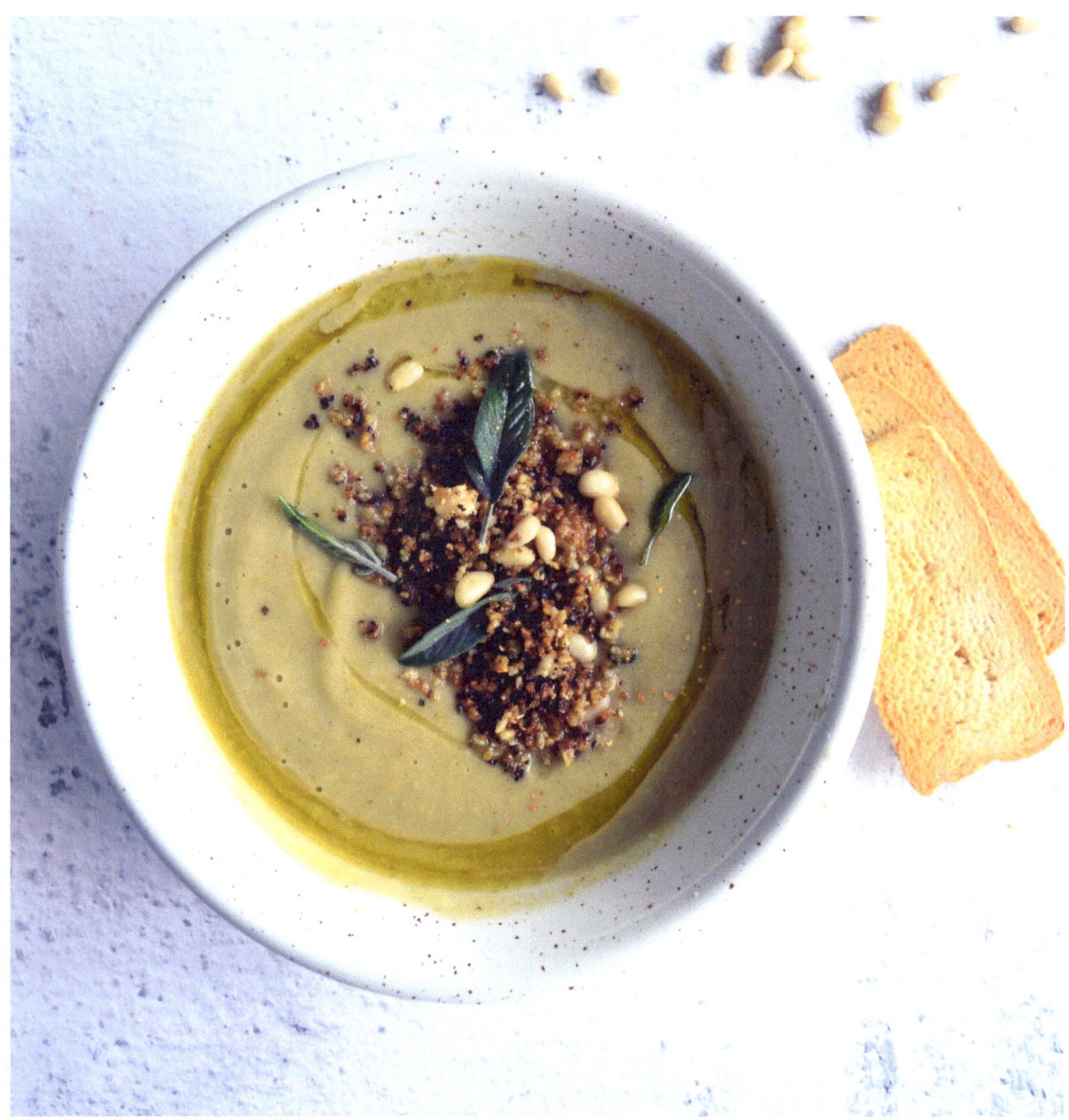

CAULIFLOWER LEEK SOUP WITH SAGE AND PINE NUTS

Time - 30 minutes
Serves - 3-4

Ingredients
1 medium head cauliflower (approx. 550 g)
2 leeks
5-6 garlic cloves
4 tbsp vegetable stock
1/4 tsp sage powder
1/4 tsp white pepper
600 ml water

Crumble
4 tbsp pine nuts
2 tbsp walnuts
1 tbsp nutritional yeast
4-5 fresh sage leaves
A pinch of salt and black pepper

1. Cut the leeks into small pieces, place in a large pan along with the garlic cloves. Add some water or vegetable stock, cook until soften.
2. Then add the cauliflower florets, cover with water. Bring to boil until soften.
3. Transfer mixture from pan to a high speed blender. Add some water depending on your blender and how liquid you like. I added 600 ml water. Season with salt, pepper and sage.
4. Blend mixture until silky smooth. Then transfer to a deep pot. Taste it, if it is too thick, then add more water and salt. Then cook for 3-4 minutes on medium heat.
5. To make the pine nut crumble, place all ingredients into a small food processor. Pulse several times until it is roughly chopped.
6. Then transfer crumble to a skillet over medium heat and gently toast the crumble, stirring constantly for about 3-4 minutes until golden and fragrant.
7. Serve your soup with crumble. Season with salt and pepper. Decorate with toasted sage leaves if desired.

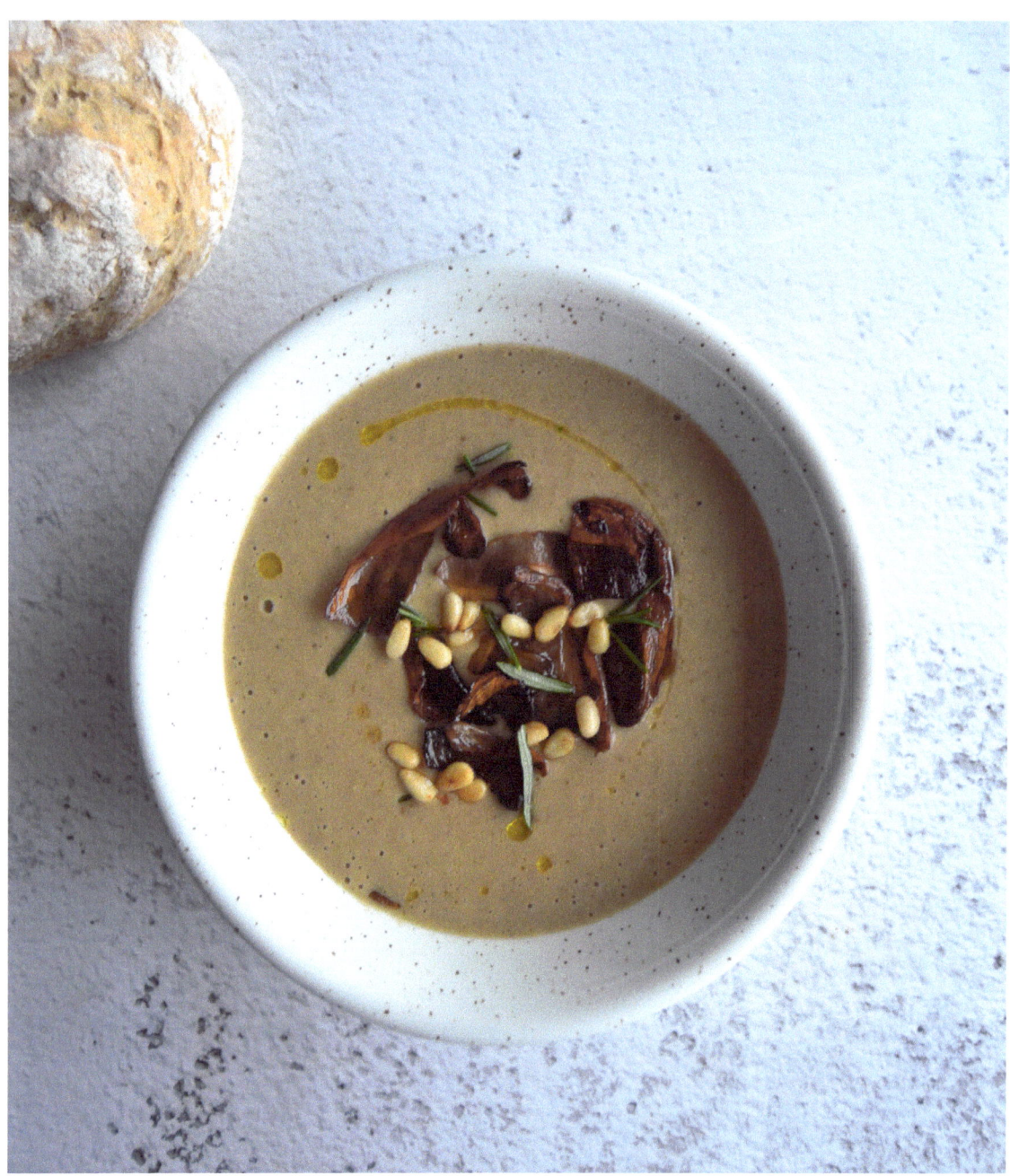

PORCINI SOUP

Time - 30 minutes
Serves - 3-4

Ingredients
40 g dried mushrooms
Mushroom stock (200ml from dried mushrooms, soak mushrooms in warm water for one hour then strain use the water in the soup)
3 tbsp olive oil
1 medium leek chopped
1 medium onion chopped
3 garlic cloves minced
Salt and pepper to taste
200 ml oat milk
1/2 tsp fresh rosemary chopped
2 tbsp toasted pine nuts

1. To a large saucepan, add the olive oil over medium-high heat. Add the mushrooms, sauté until soft and browned. Remove 1/3 of mushrooms and set aside for garnish later.

2. Add the leeks, onion, garlic salt and pepper. Continue to sauté until they are soft. Add the rosemary, cook for 2 minutes. Add oat milk and mushroom stock. Bring to a boil, reduce heat and simmer for 15 minutes.

3. Transfer mixture in to a high speed blender, mix well until completely smooth. If it is too thick add some water and continue to blender.

4. Put the soup back into the pot, add the mushrooms that were set aside. Reheat and test for seasoning, add salt if needed. Serve with toasted pine nuts.

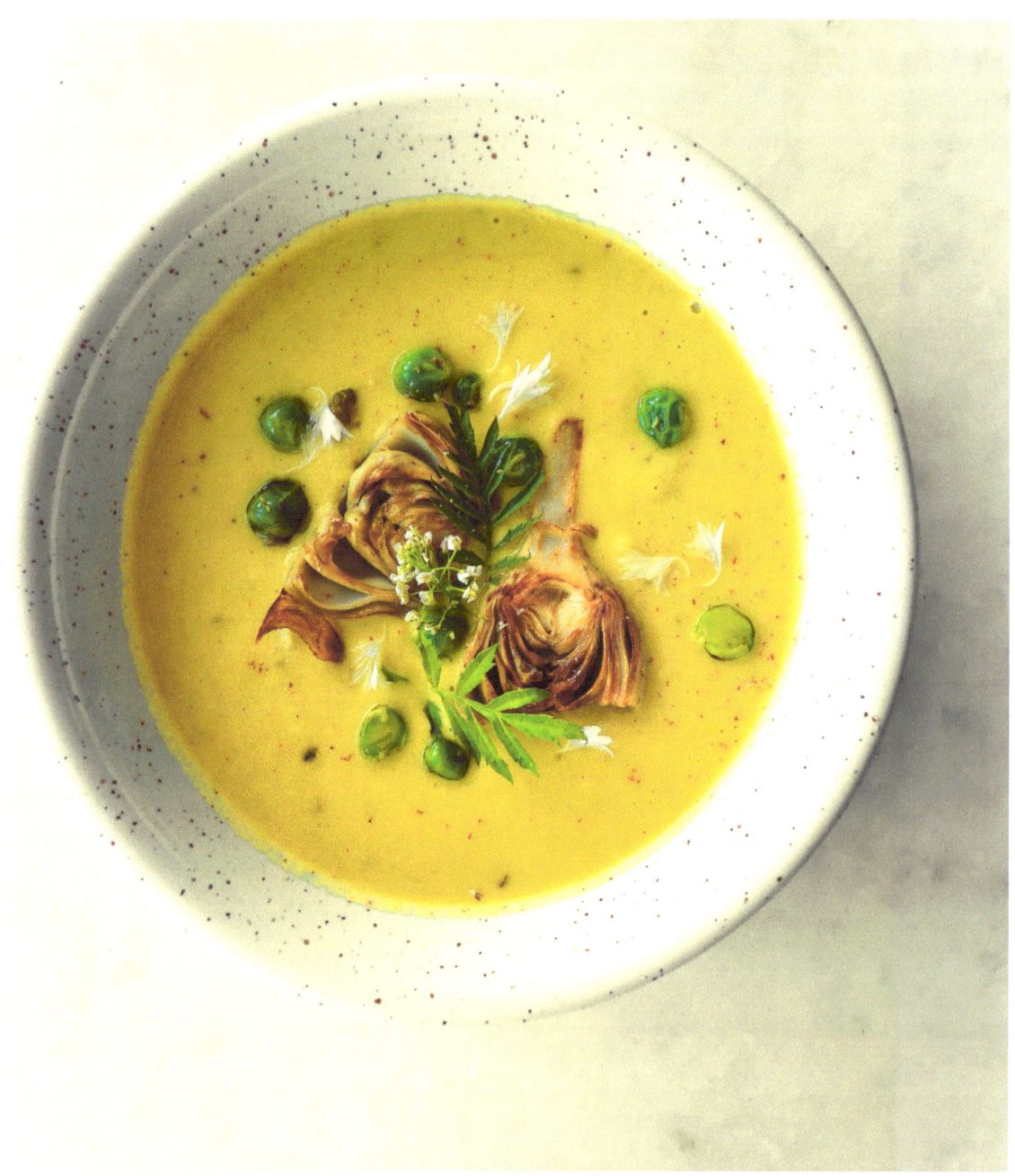

ARTICHOKE PEA SOUP

Time - 30 minutes
Serves - 3-4

Ingredients
1/2 fennel
1 large carrot
1 large onion
3 pieces of artichoke hearts (+ 2 pieces halved, pan fried for garnish)
200 g green peas
Juice of 1 lemon
1 tablespoon of olive oil
400 ml vegetable stock
Salt and pepper to taste
1/4 teaspoon nutmeg

1. Chop the onion, carrot and fennel finely. Place in a pan, drizzle olive oil. Cook for 2-3 minutes on medium-high heat until caramelized.

2. Add the pea and vegetable stock, continue to cook for 5-6 minutes.

3. Transfer the mixture to the blender. Add the lemon juice, nutmeg, salt and pepper to it. Mix until you get a smooth consistency. Add more water if necessary.

4. Transfer the soup to the pot, cook over low-medium heat.

5. Serve with pan-fried artichoke hearts and toasted peas. Garnish with edible flowers if desired.

GOURMET VEGAN

SALAD BOWLS

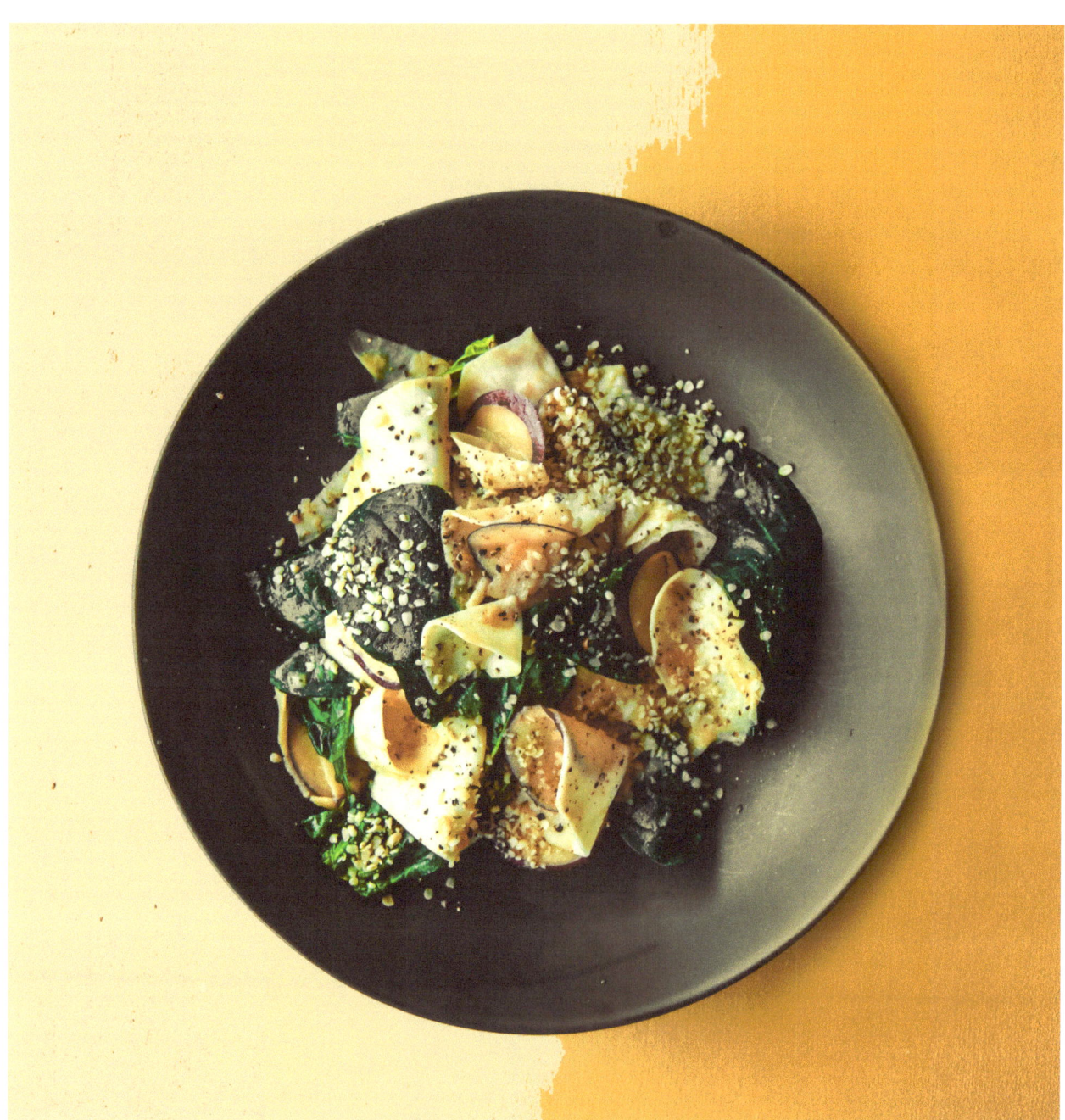

RAW CELERIAC SALAD WITH SPINACH, APPLES AND HEMP

Time - 20 minutes
Serves - 3-4

Ingredients
2 celeriac
2 red apples
2 cups baby spinach
1/4 cup hemp hearts
Blackpepper and salt to taste

Dressing
30 ml lemon juice
35 ml olive oil
2 tbsp grape molasses
2 tbsp dijon mustard
2 tbsp vegan white wine or apple cider vinegar

1. Peel the skin of your celeriac. Using a mandoline slicer, thinly slice it. Make sure you have thinly shavings. Root vegetables are very tasty and easy to eat when you slice thinly.
2. Slice apples using the mandoline as well.
3. In a large bowl, add the baby spinach, celeriac and apple shavings.
4. To make the dressing, in a bowl mix the all dressing ingredients well to combine together.
5. Pour the dressing over the celeriac, apple and spinach. Massage well using your hands.
6. Add the blackpepper, salt and hemp hearts. Toss together.
7. Let it marinate at least one hour. Then serve as a side dish or main. For a fulfilling meal, pair it with vegetable balls, rice or pasta.

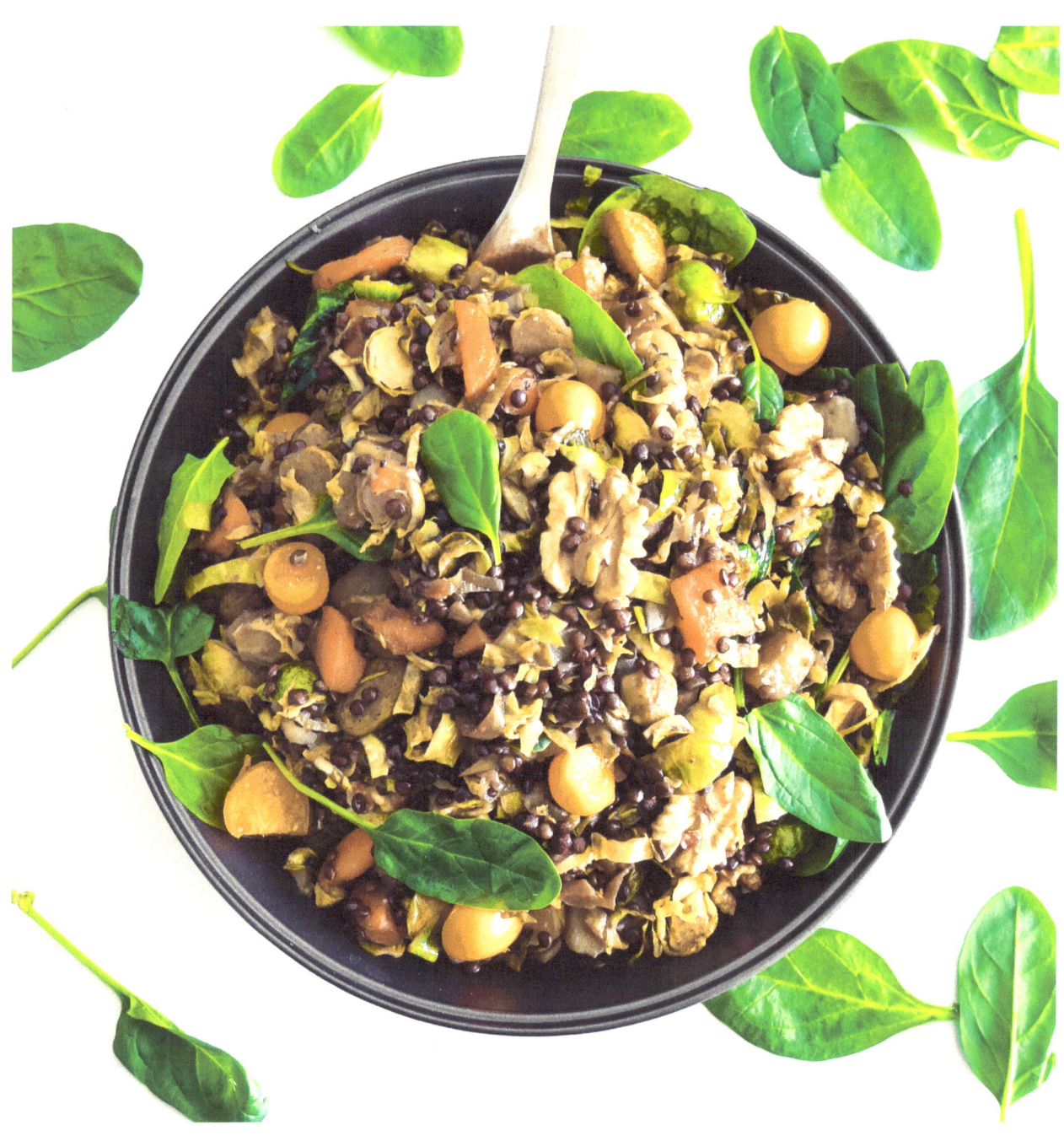

BELUGA SALAD WITH BRUSSELS SPROUTS SPINACH AND INCABERRIES

Time - 30 minutes
Serves - 3-4

Ingredients
1 leek sliced thinly
1 cup beluga lentil
2 tbsp pomegranate syrup
2 tbsp pumpkin seeds
Salt and pepper to taste
4 tbsp lemon Juice
1 tsp ginger powder
2 tbsp grape molasses
2 tbsp extra virgin olive oil
300 g brussels sprouts
A handful of walnuts
1/2 cup incaberries
2 tbsp chopped fresh rosemary
2 cups baby spinach

1. Finely chop leeks and brussel sprouts, add to a pan. On low-medium heat cook until soften stirring occasionaly. Add some water in order to prevent sticking to the pan. You can also add olive oil if desired. But scientists found that heating up vegetable oils led to the release of high concentrations of chemicals called aldehydes, which have been linked to illnesses including cancer, heart disease and dementia. So It is best to cook with water as much as we can do.

2. To make dressing, in a bowl mix pomegranate syrup, lemon juice, salt, pepper, ginger powder, grape molasses and extra virgin olive oil together. Set aside.

3. In a large bowl, add washed and drained baby spinach leaves, add cooked beluga lentil on top, add cooked brussel sprouts and leeks. Then add walnuts, fresh rosemary and halved incaberries.

4. Pour dressing over the salad. Toss well with all ingredients. Spread pumkin seeds. Divide between bowls. Taste it, adjust seasonsing if desired. Enjoy!

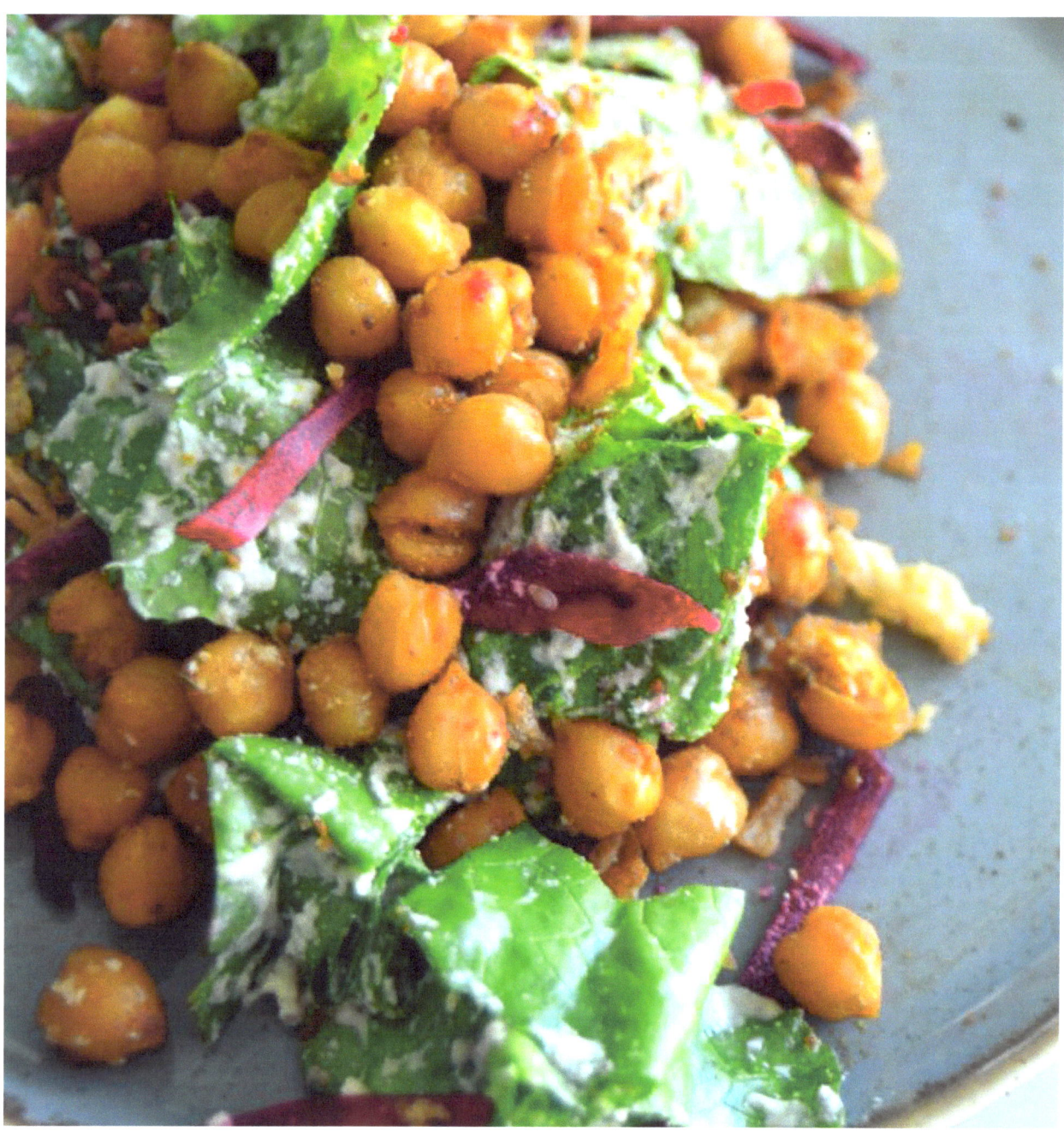

KALE WITH TOASTED CHICKPEAS AND ALMOND CREAM

Time - 40 minutes
Serves - 2-3

Salad Ingredients
1 bundle kale leaves
1 tbsp grapeseed oil
2 tbsp lemon juice
1/2 tsp salt
1 small beetroot grated
3-4 tbsp crispy fried onions

Spicy Chickpea
1 cup chickpeas
3 tbsp grapeseed oil
1 tsp dried thyme
1/2 tsp ground turmeric
1/4 tsp coriander
1/2 tsp red pepper flakes
1/4 tsp cinnamon
1/4 tsp cardamom

Ceasar Sauce
2 cloves of garlic
3-4 tablespoons lemon juice
A pinch of blackpepper
1 teaspoon dried mint
1/ tablespoon maple syrup
A pinch of sea salt
1/4 cup water to thin,
80 g raw almonds pre-soaked

1. Pre-heat oven to 200° C. In a large bowl, mix all spicy chickpea ingredients well. Add chickpeas into the bowl, stir to combine well.
2. Place a parchment paper on the baking tray. Transfer chickpeas here. Bake for 25 minutes or until crispy enough.

3. Wash and rinse kale leaves, cut into 2-3 small pieces. Place in a large bowl. Pour almond caesar sauce and massage with your hands to soften and coat the kale for about 1-2 minutes.

4. When chickpeas are baked, spread them onto the salad. Add grated beets. Spread some crispy fried onion. Add salt, lemon and juice if you need. Enjoy!

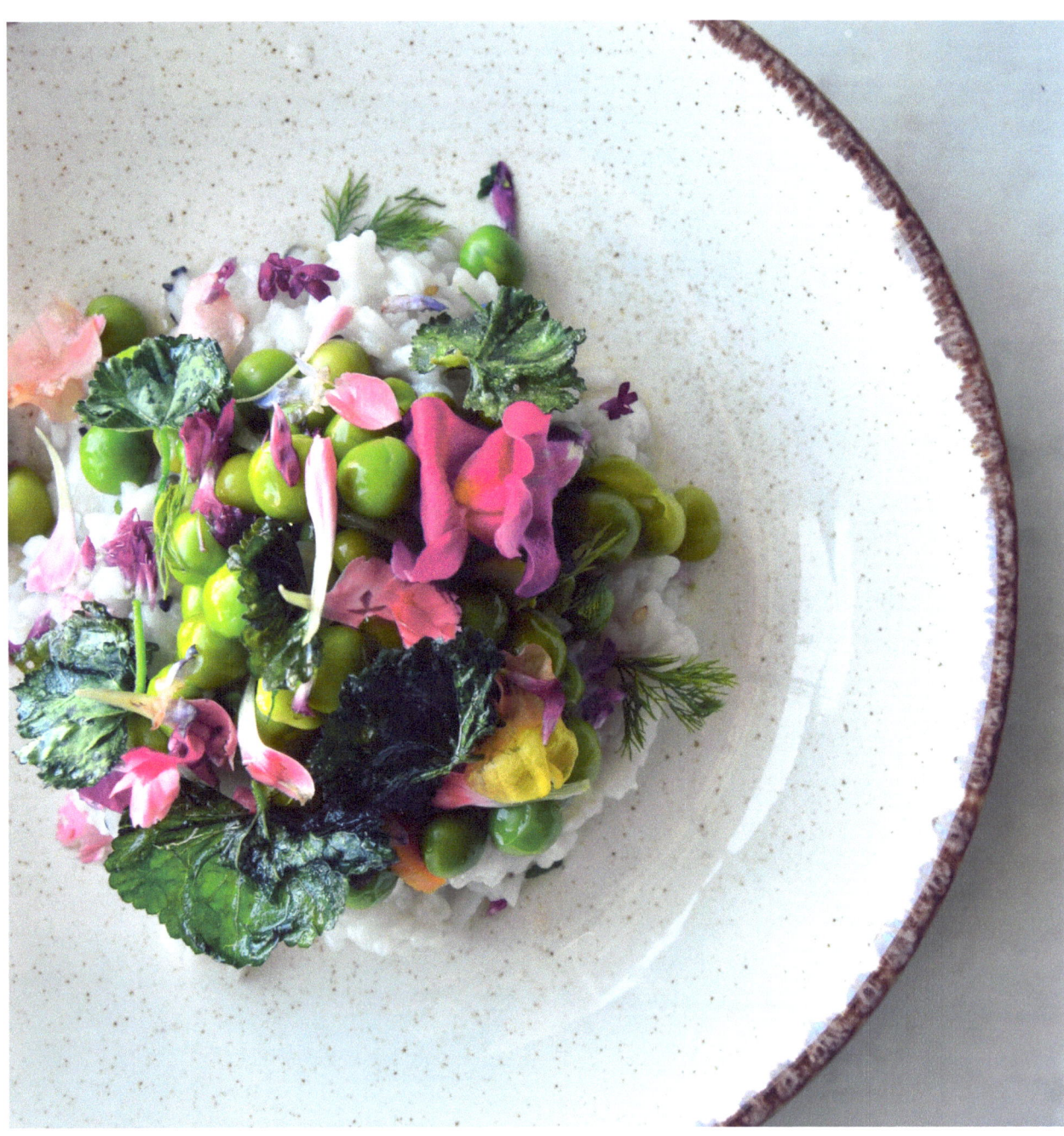

RICE WITH PEAS AND MALVA

Time - 35 minutes
Serves - 2-3

Ingredients
1 cup rice of your choice
1/2 cup green peas
2 tbsp olive oil
Salt and blackpepper to taste
1/2 cup malve leaves (or collard, spinach, kale, mustard greens etc.)
1/4 cup chopped fresh dill
2 tbsp lemon juice
Edible flowers for garnish (optional)

1. Wash and cook your rice according to package instructions.

2. Set aside to let it cool for 15 minutes.

3. Meanwhile add the green peas on a pan, toss with 1 tbsp olive oil until toasted well. Set aside.

4. Add the another tbsp olive oil and malva leaves on the pan, toss together and fry until crispy.

5. Serve your rice with toasted green peas, crispy malva leaves, lemon juice and edible flowers. Adjust the salt and pepper.

SALAD BOWLS

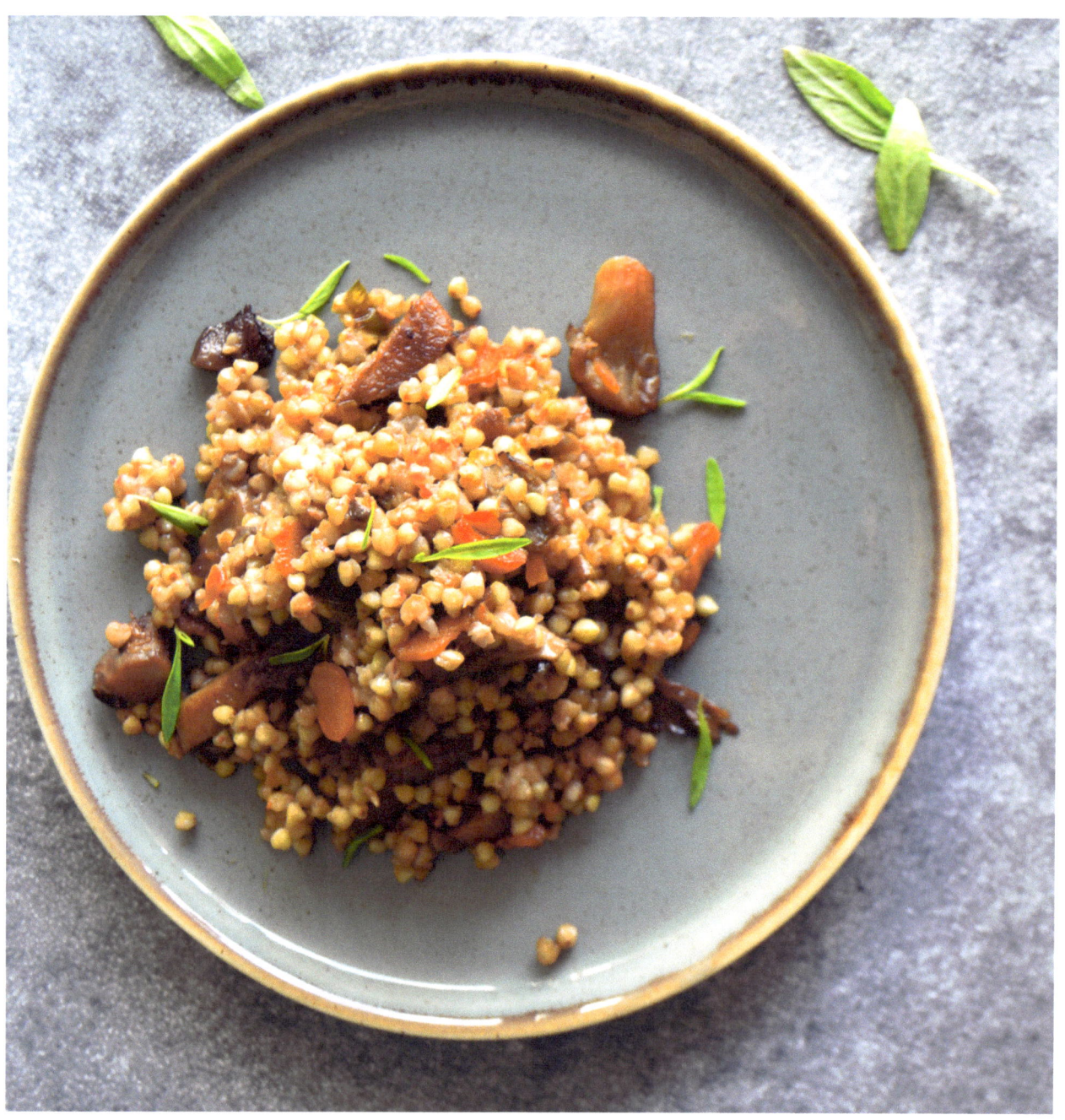

BUCKOTTO WITH MUSHROOMS

Time - 40 minutes
Serves - 2

Ingredients
400 g mushrooms of your choice
100 g buckwheat
100 ml water
1 medium red onion chopped
2 garlic cloves minced
2 tbsp tamari or soy sauce
125 ml oat cream or plant-based cream of your choice
2 tbsp olive oil
1 red bell pepper
1 green pepper
Fresh tarragon to serve (optional)
1 tsp sesame seeds
1 tsp salt

1. Brush your mushrooms to clean and slice them thinly.

2. Cut peppers into small pieces. In a large skillet add the olive oil, peppers and onion. Stir-fry on high heat for 2 minutes.

3. Then add the mushroom slices, soy sauce, thyme, salt and garlic powder. Cook on medium heat until browned and tendered.

4. Add the oat cream and cook for 5 minutes.

5. In a small pot, place the buckwheats. Cover with water and bring to boil for 20 minutes or until lightly soften. Then remove, strain and transfer them into the skillet. Mix with mushrooms well.

6. Decorate with parsley or your favorite herbs.

SALAD BOWLS

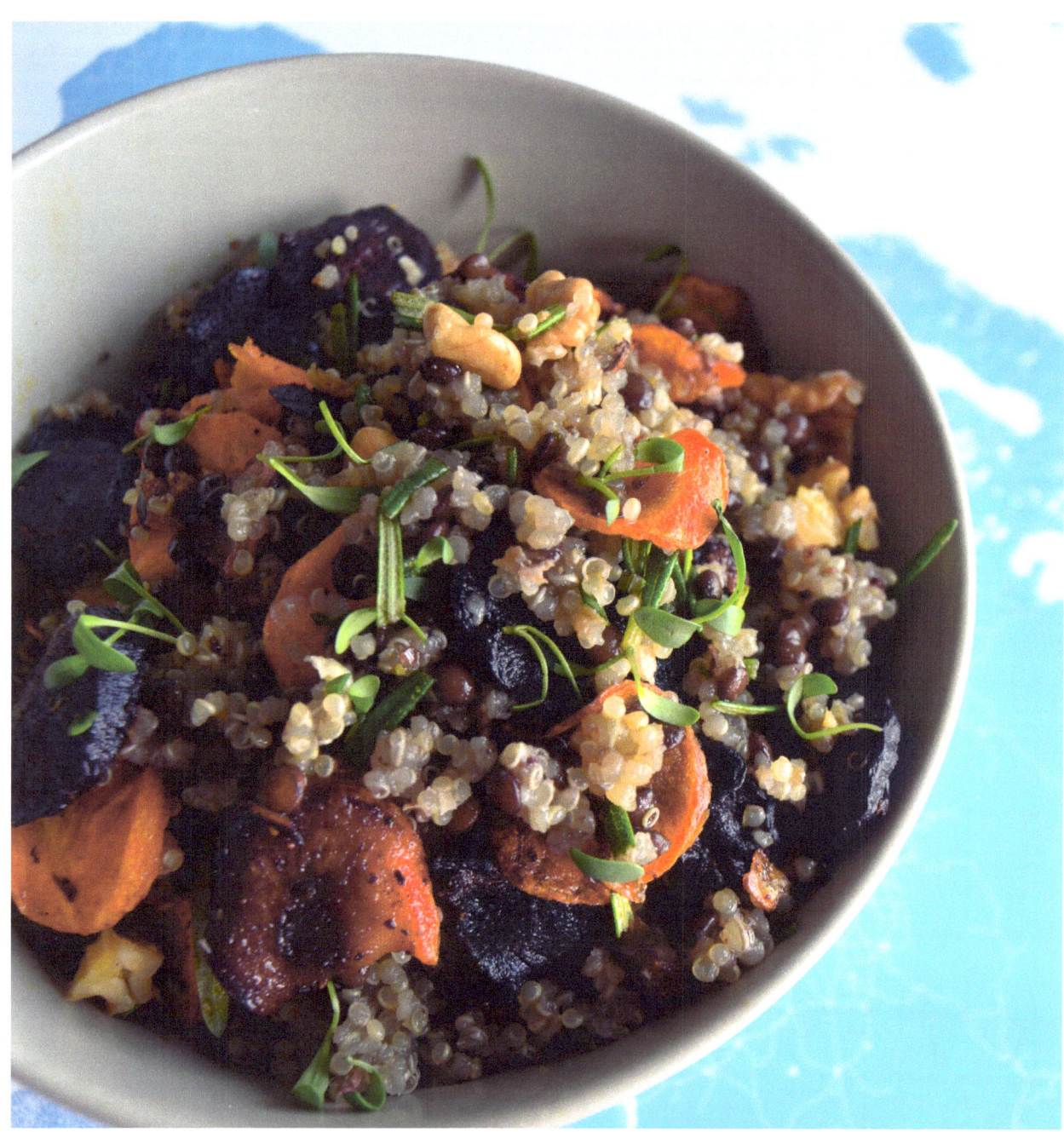

CHILI CARROT QUINOA

Time - 30 minutes
Serves - 3-4

Ingredients
1/2 cup quinoa cooked
1/4 cup beluga lentil cooked
2 colorful carrots
1 red onion thinly sliced
1 tsp garlic powder or minced garlic
1 tsp turmeric powder
1 tsp paprika
1/2 cup chopped walnuts
Salt and peppper to taste
3-4 tbsp olive oil
Microgreens to serve
1 tsp chili sauce

1. Pre-heat oven to 200° C, line a tray with parchment paper. Set aside cooked quinoa and beluga lentil. Cut carrots and onions thinly. Mix the rest of the ingredients except walnuts, microgreens and rosemary together. Then coat carrots with the sauce well.

2. Spread veggies onto baking tray evenly and roast for about 25 minutes. Place cooked quinoa and beluga lentil in a bowl, add walnuts, salt and pepper. Toss together.

3. When carrots are baked, then add into the bowl, mix with quinoa mixture. Drizzle some olive oil if you need. Give it a good toss and serve with micro greens.

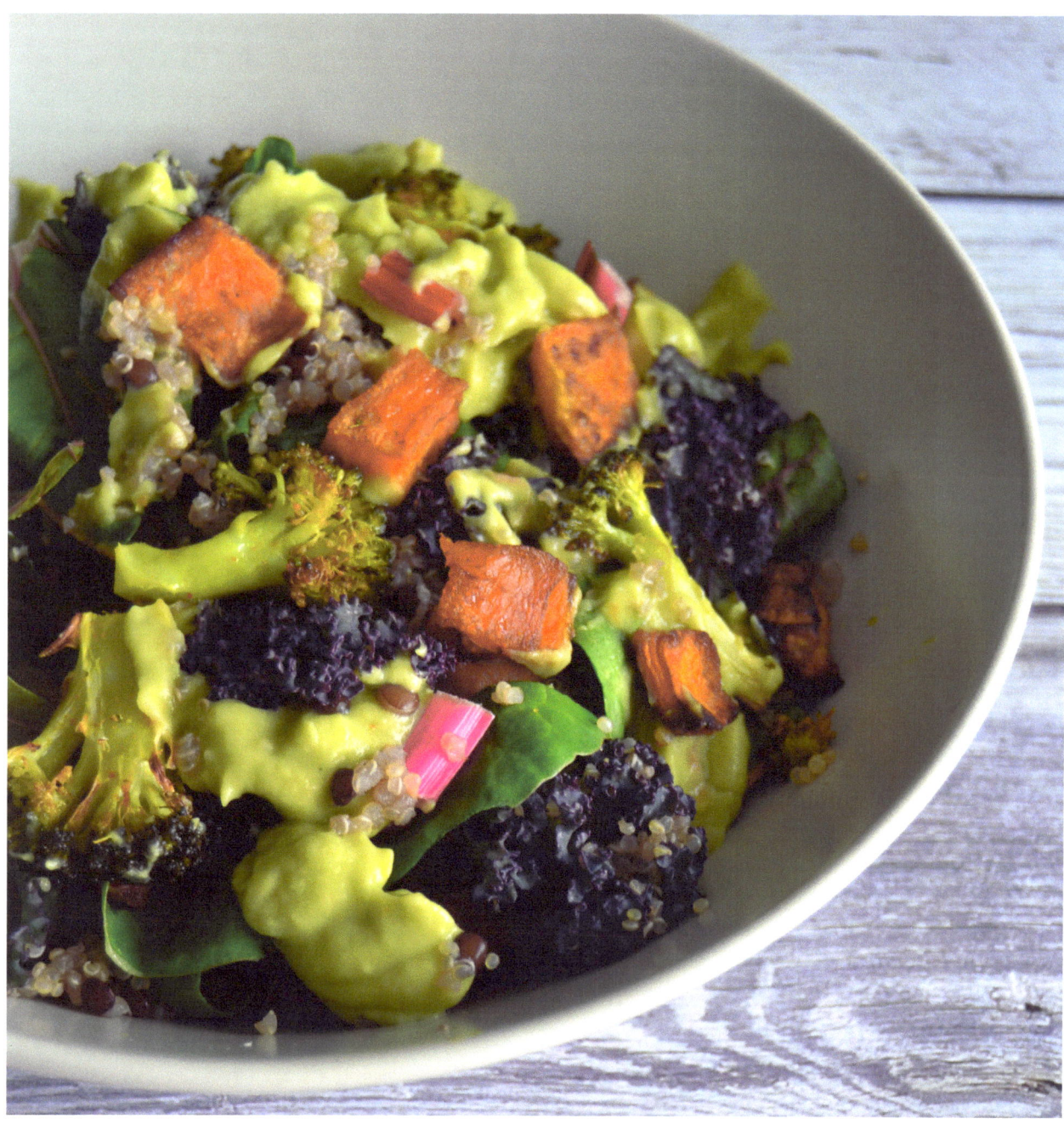

ROASTED VEGGIE QUINOA SALAD

Time - 35 minutes
Serves - 2

Ingredients
100 g butternut squash
1 broccoli head
1 tsp turmeric
Salt and pepper to taste
50 g beluga lentil cooked
100 g kale chopped
2 large leaves of swiss chard
1 tsp sesame seeds

Avocado Dressing
1 ripe avocado
1/2 lemon juice
1/8 tsp salt
3-4 cherry tomatoes
1 Small garlic minced
1/3 tsp ground mustard
1 small jalapeno

1. Pre-heat the oven to 200° C and place a parchment paper to a large roasting tray and add the olive oil. Add the butternut squash and toss in the oil. Roast for 10 minutes. Cut broccoli heads into small florets. Then add the broccoli with the spices, salt and pepper. Roast for a further 20 minutes.

2. Meanwhile, add the cooked quinoa and lentils to a large bowl and mix in the kale and swiss chard leaves. Once the veggies are cooked and cooled slightly, mix into the salad with the leaves, quinoa and lentils.

3. Place all sauce ingredients into the food processor, mix on high speed. Pour over the salad. Sprinkle sesame seeds.

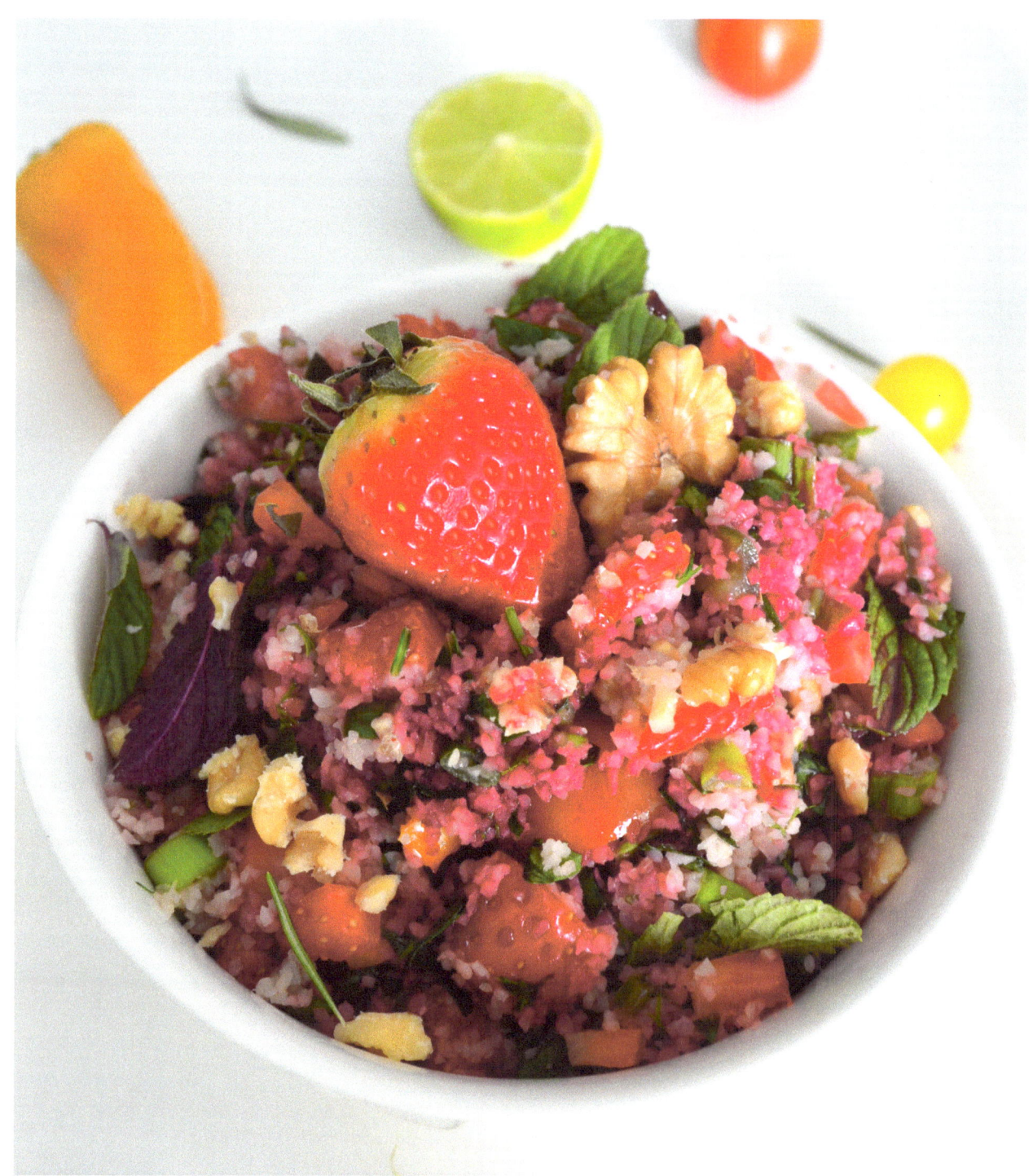

SWEET TEMPEST TABOULLEH BOWL

Time - 20 minutes
Serves - 2-3

Ingredients
200 g fine bulgur
1/2 cup cherry tomatoes
1 red bell pepper
1 yellow capsicum
1/2 bunch parsley
1/2 bunch dill
1/4 bunch mint
2 tbsp lemon juice
1/2 bunch green onion
1/2 cup strawberries
1-2 tbsp pomegranate syrup

1. Wash your bulgur well, strain and set aside. Dice your peppers and tomatoes, chop the dill, onion and parsley finely. Place everything in a large mixing bowl.

2. Transfer bulgur into the bow, toss well together.

3. Add the lemon juice, salt, walnuts, strawberries and pomegranate syrup. Give it a good toss again.

4. Serve cold for the best result.

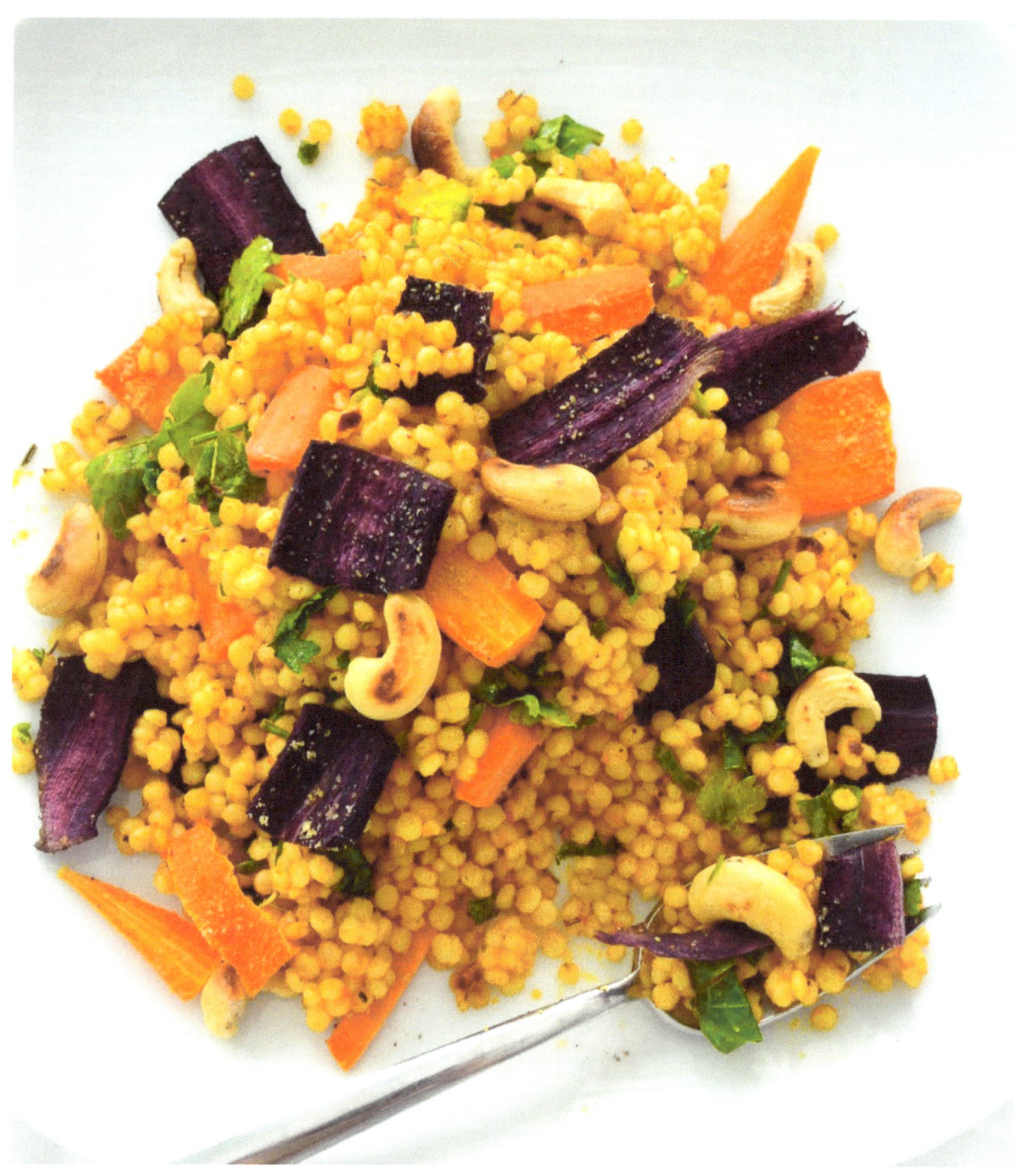

COUSCOUS WITH CARROTS AND TOASTED CASHEWS

Time - 45 minutes

Serves - 2-3

Ingredients
3 colorful carrots
1 cup couscous
40 g cashews
1/2 bunch parsley
2 tbsp olive oil
1 tsp paprika
1/2 tsp chipotle
1 tsp turmeric
1 tsp dijon mustard
1 tsp chopped fresh rosemary
1/4 cup chopped greens of your choice
Salt and pepper to taste

1. Pre-heat the oven to 220° C. Peel and chop the carrots, place in a roasting pan and toss with 1 tablespoon of oil, ground mustard and garlic powder. Spread out in an even layer and roast in the oven at least 20 minutes.

2. Wash and strain couscous, cover with water and cook for 10-15 minutes. Drain and set aside to cool. Place the cashew nuts in a pan and cook them over medium heat for a few minutes until golden brown. Make sure you stir often as they can burn easily.

3. Mix carrots, couscous, chopped parsley and the cashews together and dress with the remaining tablespoon of olive oil, other herbs, mustard sauce and lemon juice. Serve warm!

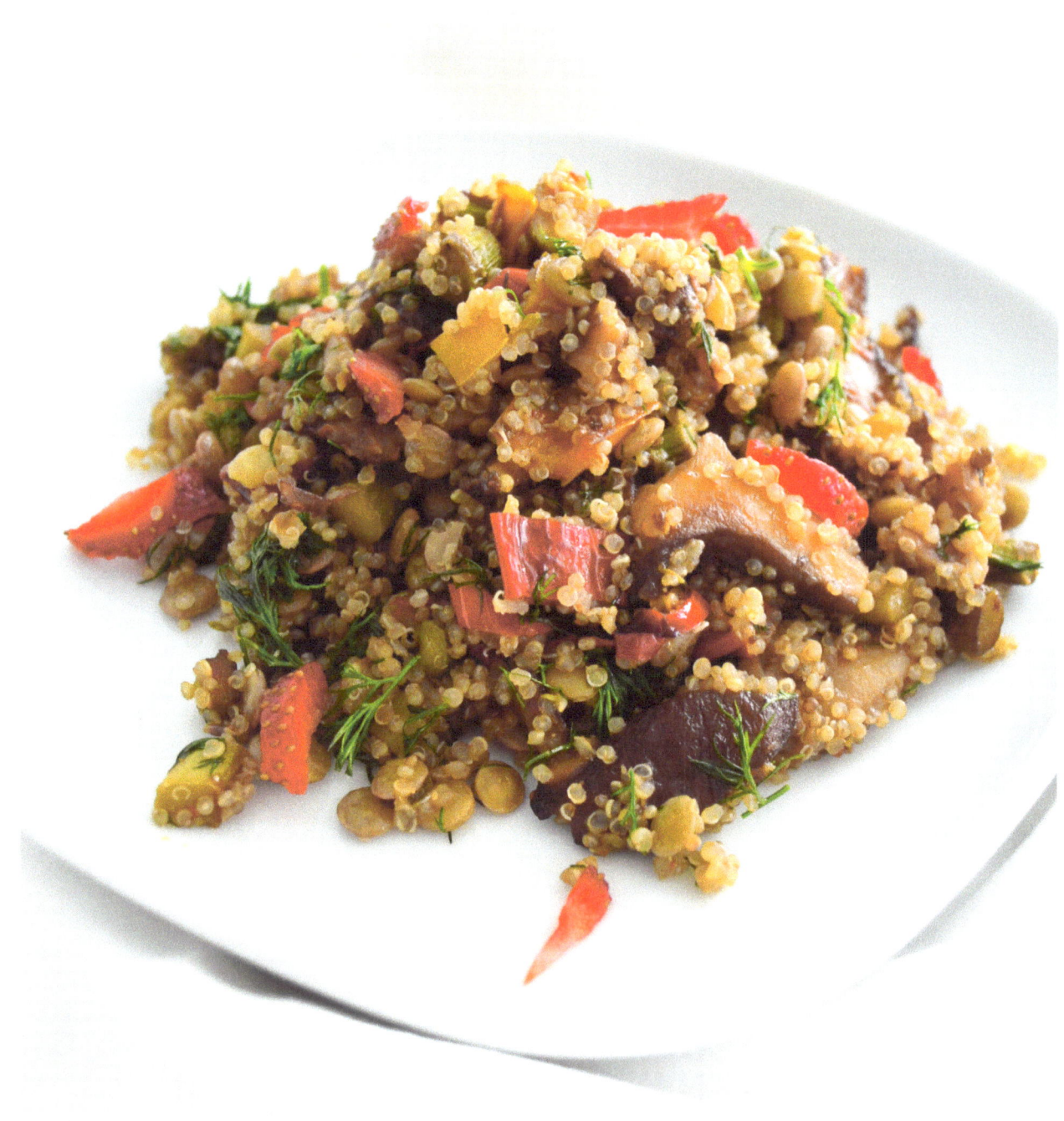

SHIITAKE QUINOA LENTIL SALAD

Time - 40 minutes
Serves - 3-4

Ingredients
100 g shiitake mushrooms
1/2 cup strawberries
2 tsp chili
5-6 asparagus stalks
1 leek
1/2 bunch fresh dill
1/2 cup quinoa
1/4 cup green lentil
2 tbsp soy sauce
1 tbsp olive oil
1/2 tsp mustard powder
3-4 tbsp lime juice

1. Place the quinoa and green lentils in a pot, cover with water. Bring to boil on medium heat for 20 minutes.

2. In a large pan, add the olive oil and soy sauce. Sauté sliced shiitakes, asparagus, leek and chili peppers on high heat stirring constantly.

3. When veggies are sautéed then add the garlic powder, thyme, mustard powder, mix well.

4. When quinoa lentil mixture are cooked, strain the excess water if you have and add to the pan. Mix with the veggies and cook for 2- 4 minutes.

5. Add the chopped strawberries and fresh dill over the salad. Give it a good toss. Serve warm with lime juice if desired.

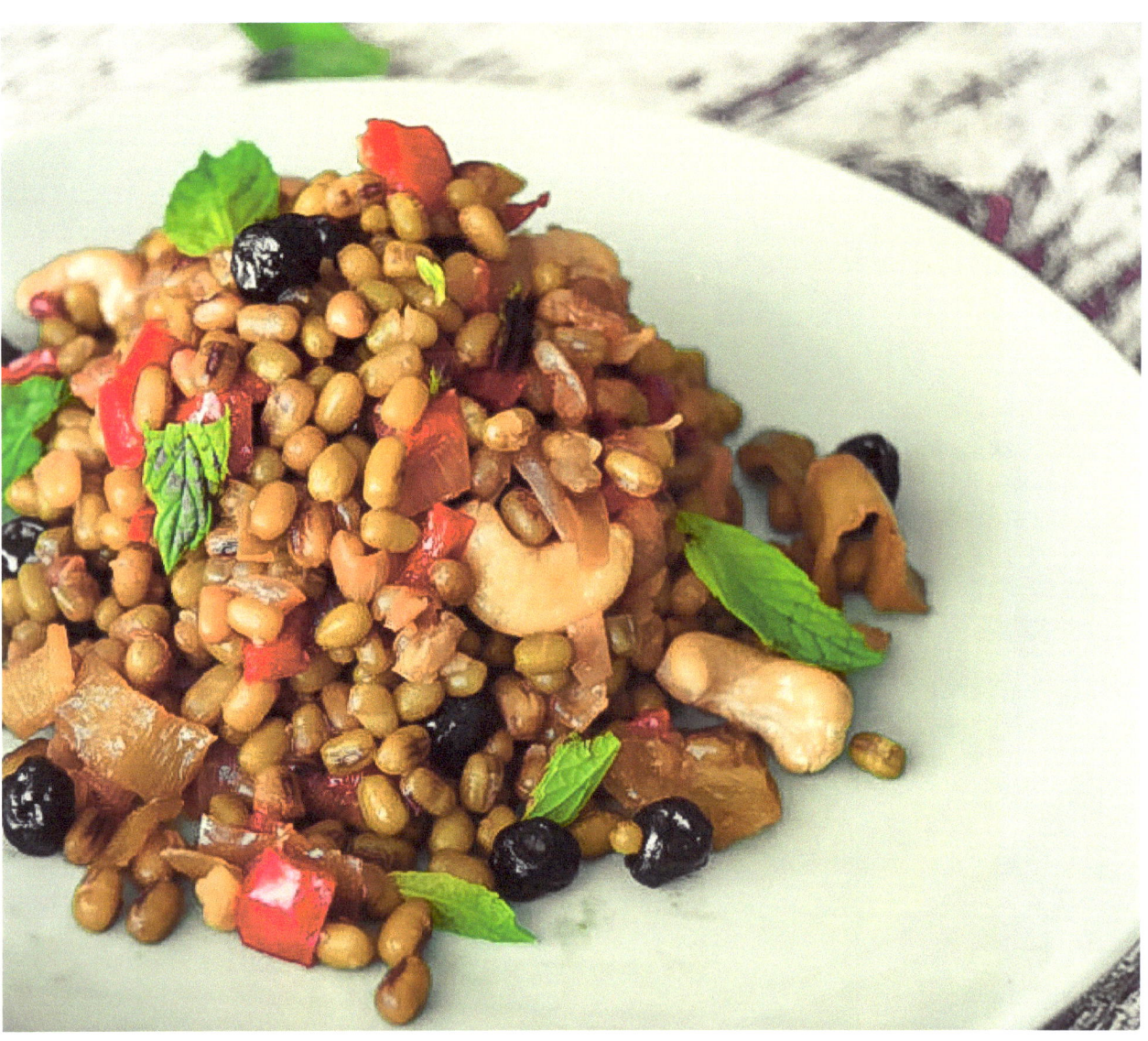

MUNG BEAN WITH BLUEBERRIES

Time - 40 minutes
Serves - 3-4

Ingredients
1 cup mung beans
1 onion chopped
1 tsp sea salt
A handful of cashews or almonds
1/2 bunch parsley
1 yellow capsicum
1 red bell pepper
2 tbsp tamari or soy sauce
1 tbsp grape molasses or maple
1 cup tangerine juice
50 g dried blueberries

1. Wash mung beans and strain. Place into a large pot, cover with water. Bring to boil on medium heat for 20 minutes or until lightly soften.

2. Saute sliced onions in the olive oil or water (if you are avoiding to heat oil). Cut peppers into very small pieces, add to the pan. Add the maple syrup, tangerine juice, cashews, blueberries, tamari, and salt. Cook on medium heat until caramelized well.

3. When mung beans are soften, add them into the pan. Occasionally stirring, cook on medium heat for about 3-4 minutes. Sprinkle fresh mint leaves or parsley on top. Serve cold or warm!

SALAD BOWLS

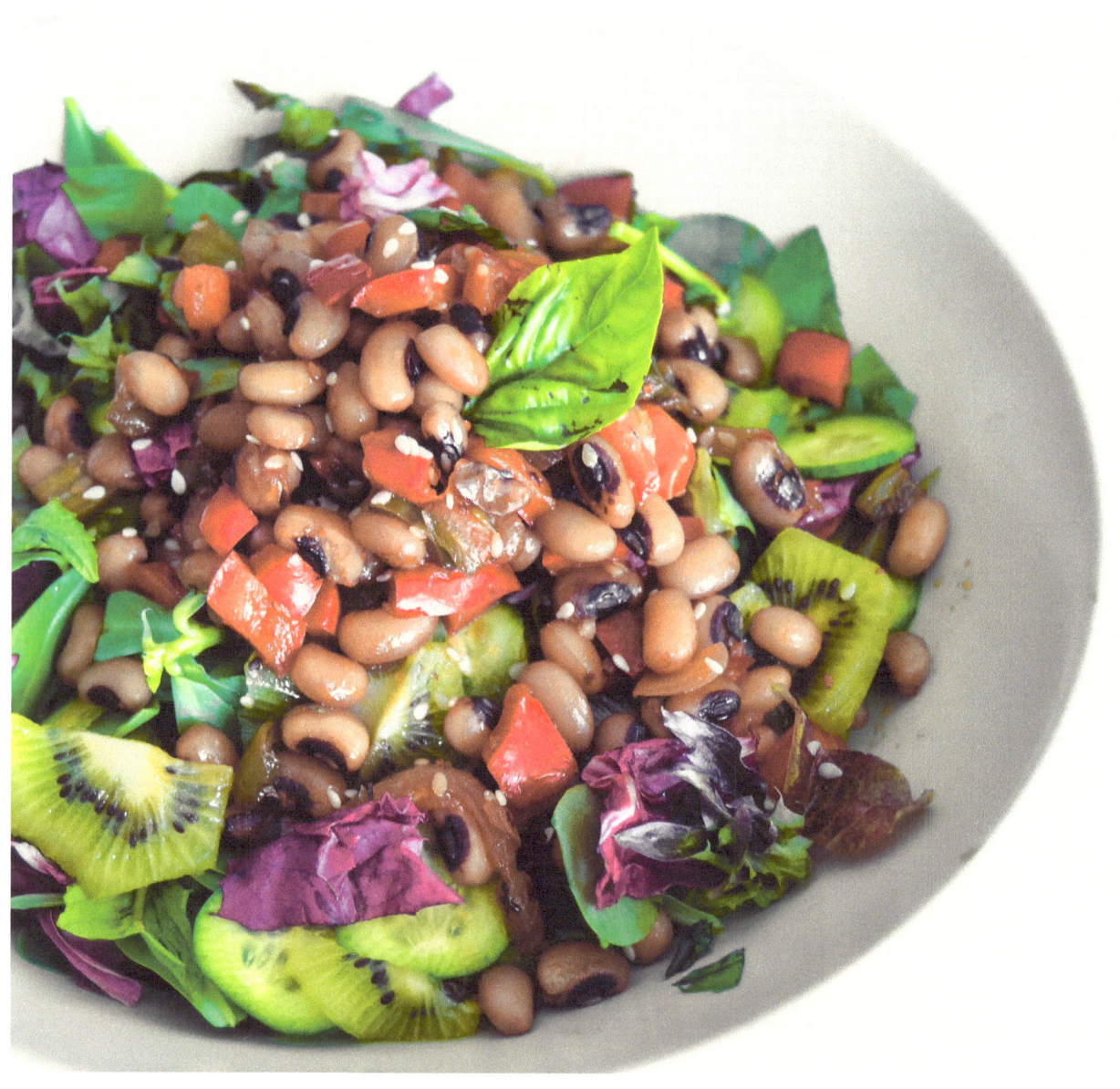

PROVENCAL COWPEA SALAD WITH KIWI

Time - 40 minutes
Serves - 3-4

Ingredients
100 g cowpeas
200 g provence greens
4 tbsp olive oil
1 onion chopped
2 tbsp tamari
1/4 tsp dried rosemary
1/4 tsp dried thyme
1/8 tsp dried mint
3 jalapeno thinly sliced
6-7 kiwi thinly sliced
1/2 cup tomatoes
2 tbsp pomegranate syrup

1. Place peas in a pot, cover with water by 2-3 inches. Bring to boil on low heat until peas are tender, but not mushy. After 20-30 minutes, strain the peas and set aside.

2. Chop your greens, thinly, slice the onion and peppers, cut kiwi slices into small chunks, divide tomatoes in halves.

3. Cut the the provence salad greens with a bamboo knife and place in a large mixing bowl. (Provencal salad is a mixture of chervil, arugula, leafy lettuces and endive in equal proportions.)

4. Add the olive oil, garlic, chopped jalapeño, onion and tamari in a pan on medium heat. Cook them for 4-5 minutes until they are soften.

5. Add the parsley, rosemary, thyme, mint, dill, lime juice and salt, stir on high heat for 1-2 minutes. Pour the beans into the pan and mix with caramelized vegetables.

6. Add the beans on top of the greens.

7. Add the pickles and tomatoes. Pour the dressing made with lime juice, pomegranate syrup and olive oil. Serve with sliced kiwis.

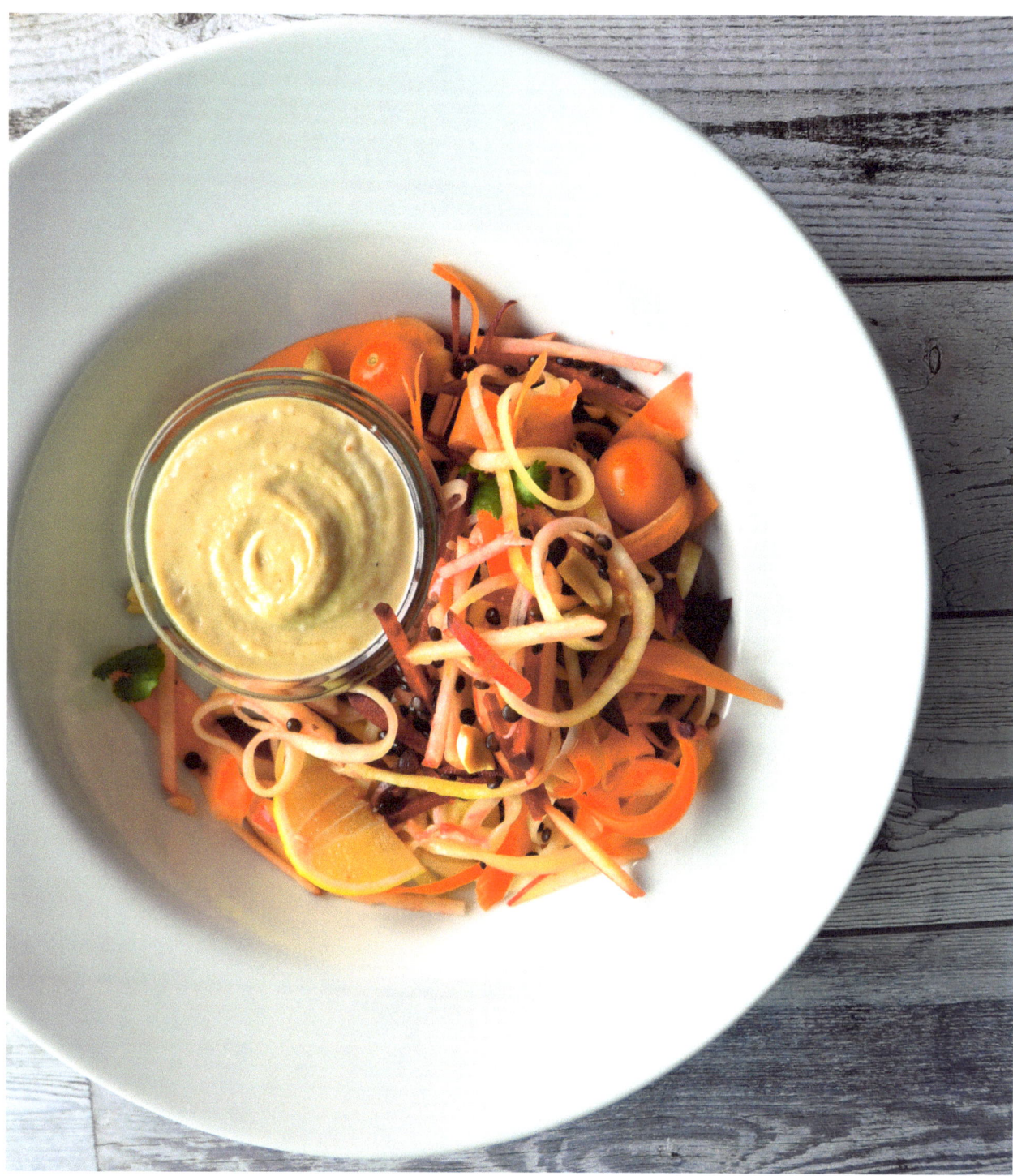

ZUCCHINI, BELUGA, APPLE SALAD WITH TAHINI DRESSING

Time - 20 minutes
Serves - 2-3

Ingredients
2 zucchini
1 carrot
1 red apple
1 small beetroot
1/4 cup cherry tomatoes
1/4 bunch cilantro or parsley
4 tbsp lemon juice
1/4 cup beluga lentils cooked or sprouted
A handful peanuts

Dressing
2 tbsp tahini
1 tbsp lemon juice
1 tbsp maple syrup
1/8 tsp salt
1/8 tsp garlic powder
Water to thin

1. Using a spiralizer spiralize thel carrots, apples and beets thinly. Cook beluga lentils for about 15 minutes. Strain and let it cool.

2. Mix and place thinly cutted vegetables into the plate. Spread peanuts and beluga lentils. Decorate with cilantro. Serve with tahini sauce and lemon.

3. In a small bowl mix tahini sauce ingredients well. Pour over the salad.

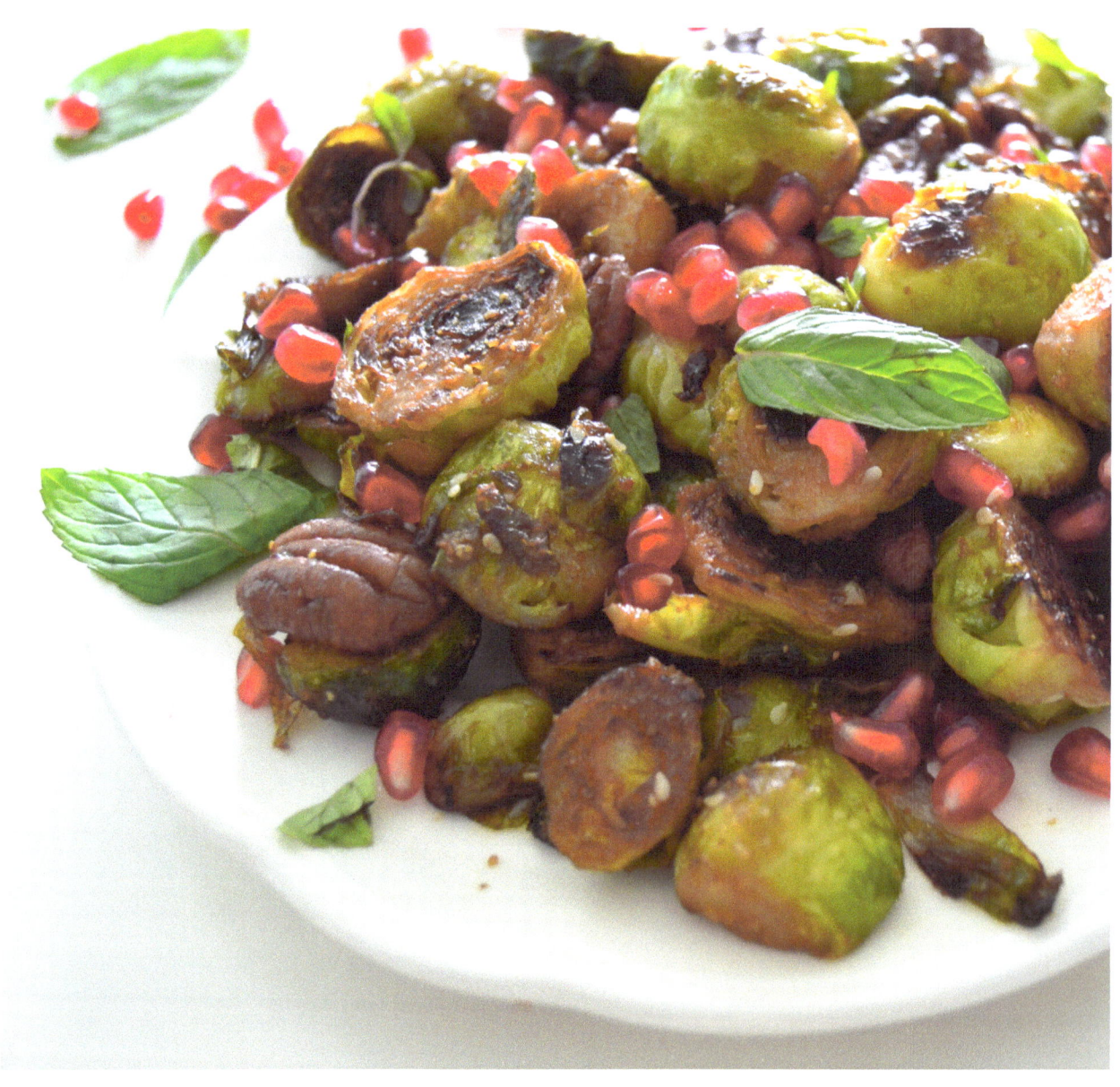

MAPLE FRIED BRUSSELS SPROUTS WITH POMEGRANATES AND PECAN

Time - 20 minutes
Serves - 2-3

Ingredients
150 g brussels sprouts
2 tbsp pomegranate syrup
2 tbsp olive oil
2 tbsp maple syrup
1 tbsp balsamic vinegar
1 tsp mustard powder
1 tsp garlic powder
1/2 cup pomegranates
1/2 cup pecan nuts toasted
1/4 cup fresh basil

1. In a large wok pan, heat oil, add halved brussel sprouts and a little bit water approx. 2-3 tbsp), cook on medium heat until lightly fried.

2. Then add balsamic vinegar, mustard powder, sea salt, garlic powder, stir well for 2-3 minutes on high heat or fried well.

3. When brussels sprouts are fried, add the pomegranate syrup and maple syrup, toss with brussels sprouts and toasted pecans. Place them in a plate, spread pomegranate seeds over the plate. Decorate with fresh basil.

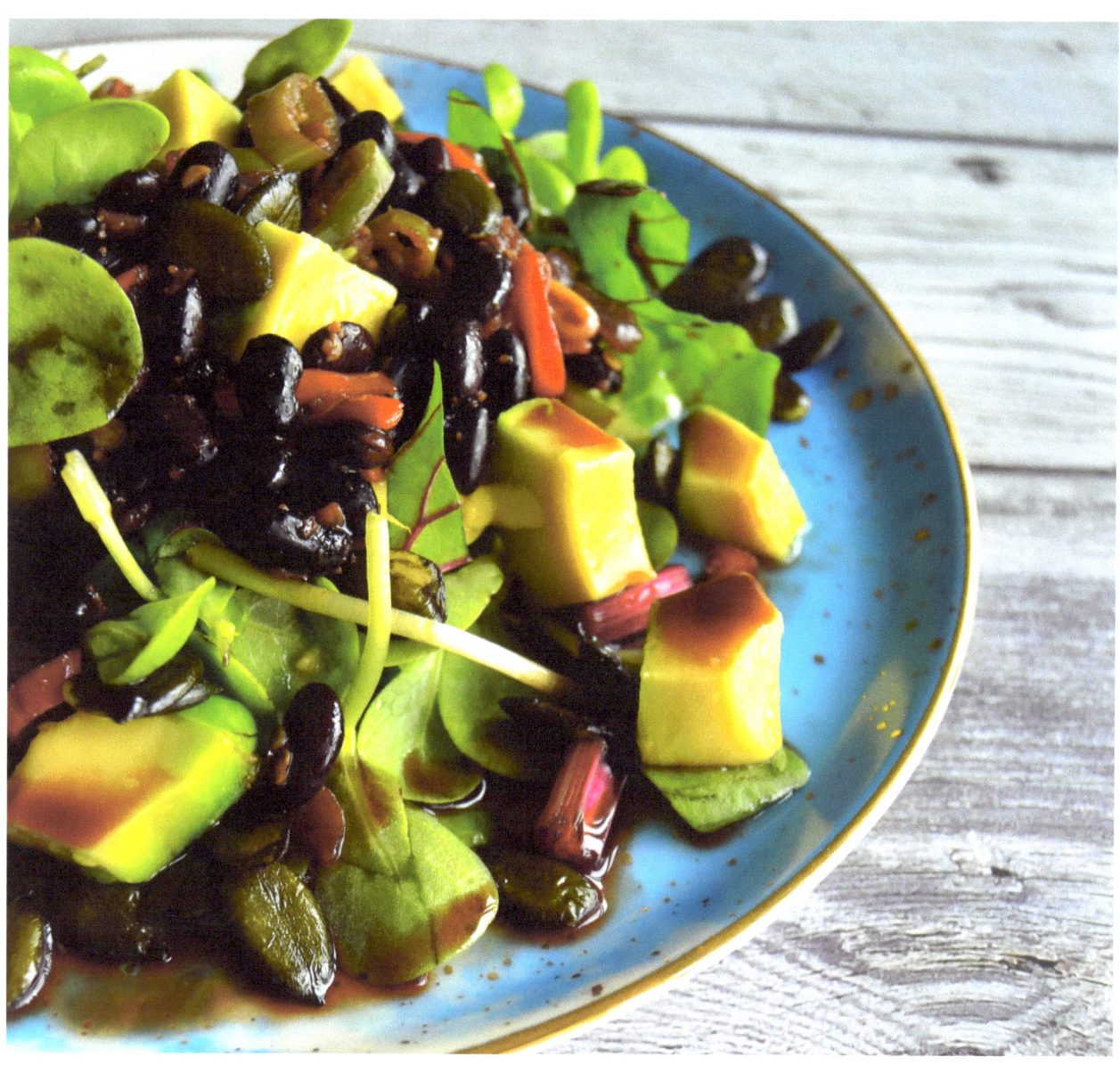

PURSLANE, AVOCADO, BEAN SALAD

Time - 20 minutes
Serves - 2-3

Ingredients
200 g purslane
1 ripe avocado
1/2 cup black beans precooked
4 tbsp pumpkin seeds
2 tbsp lemon juice
3 tbsp soy sauce or tamari
1 tsp sea salt
1 small onion chopped
1 red bell pepper chopped
1 yellow capsicum chopped
1 tsp ground mustard
1 tbsp olive oil
1 tsp garlic powder
1 tbsp balsamic

1. Wash, strain and dry purslane, set aside.

2. Peel, remove the seed of avocado and slice into cubes. Toss with lemon juice and sprinkle salt. Set aside.

3. Wash and strain your beans. Cover with filtered water, bring to boil for 30 minutes or until soften. In a large skillet pan, heat the olive oil, add the chopped onions, peppers and cook until soften, then add ground mustard, garlic powder and soy sauce. Transfer beans into the skillet. Cook on medium heat for 4-5 minutes.

4. Place the purslane into the bowl, add the beans and avocado slices. Drizzle with balsamic vinegar, sprinkle some pumpkin seeds. Serve warm or cold.

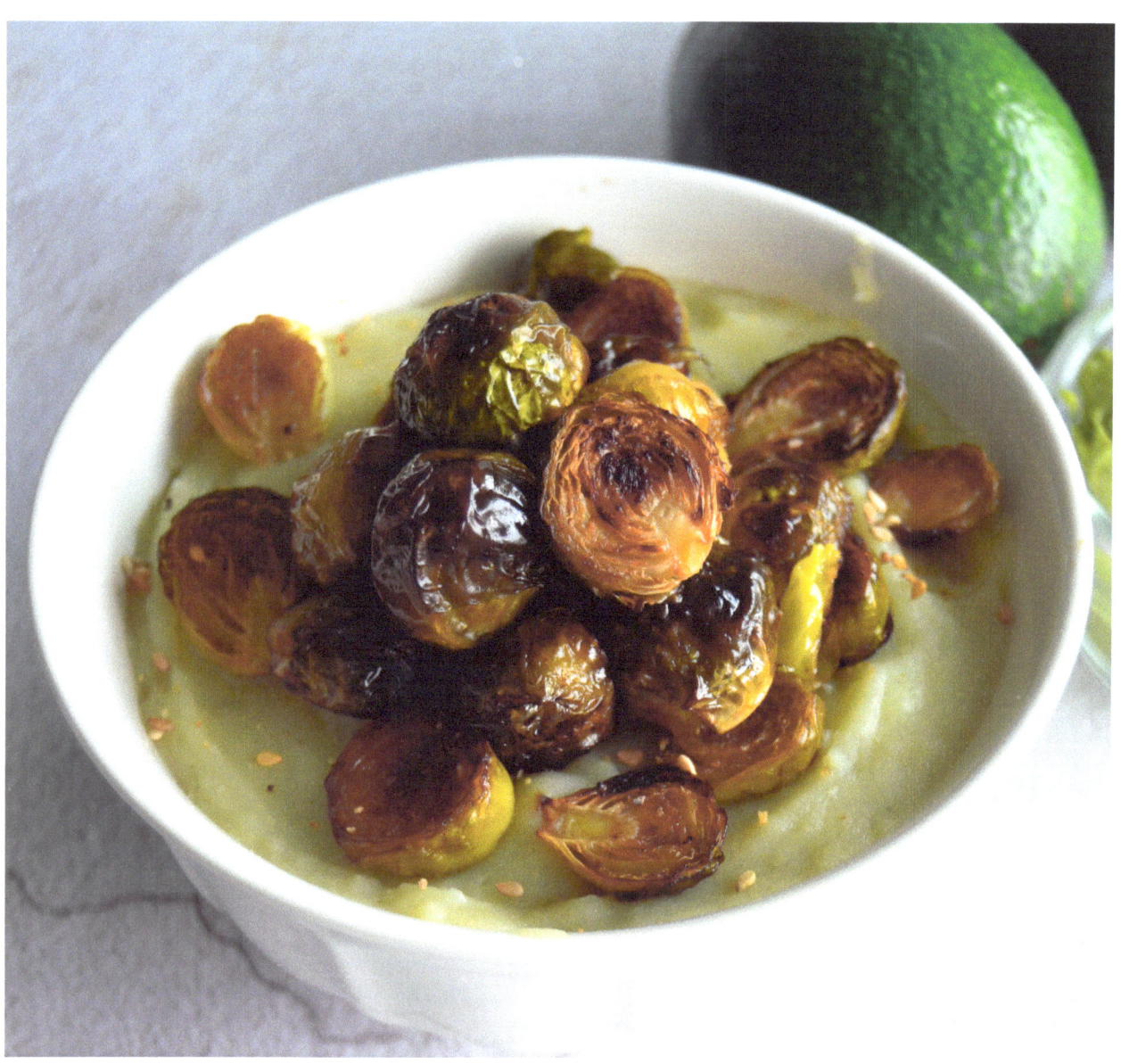

MASHED POTATO WITH BRUSSELS SPROUTS & AVOCADO

Time - 40 minutes
Serves - 3-4

Ingredients
300 g potatoes
200 g brussels sprouts
2 tbsp olive oil
1 tsp garlic powder
2 tbsp almond milk
1 tsp sea salt
1/4 tsp blackpepper

Avocado Sauce
1 ripe avocado
1 tbsp lemon juice
1/4 cup fresh basil
A handful of raw walnuts
1/4 tsp provence herbs

1. Wash, drain and cut brussels sprouts in halves. Drizzle with olive oil and bake in the oven at 200° C until golden.

2. Place the potatoes in a large pot, cover with cold water. Add a little salt in to the water. Over high heat, bring the water to a boil, then reduce heat to maintain a low boil. Cook for about 25-30 minutes or until potatoes are very tender.

3. Drain potatoes well and remove the skin. Place them in a food processor, add almond milk, salt & pepper. Mix on high speed until smooth and creamy. Add an additional tablespoons of almond milk if you need. But be careful, because too much milk can make the potatoes soupy. ttransfer potatoes into a bowl, add baked brussels sprouts on top.

4. To make avocado sauce, place fresh basil, lemon juice, salt, avocado and walnut into the food processor, mix on high speed until smooth.
Transfer in a small bowl. Serve with mashed potatoes and baked brussel sprouts.

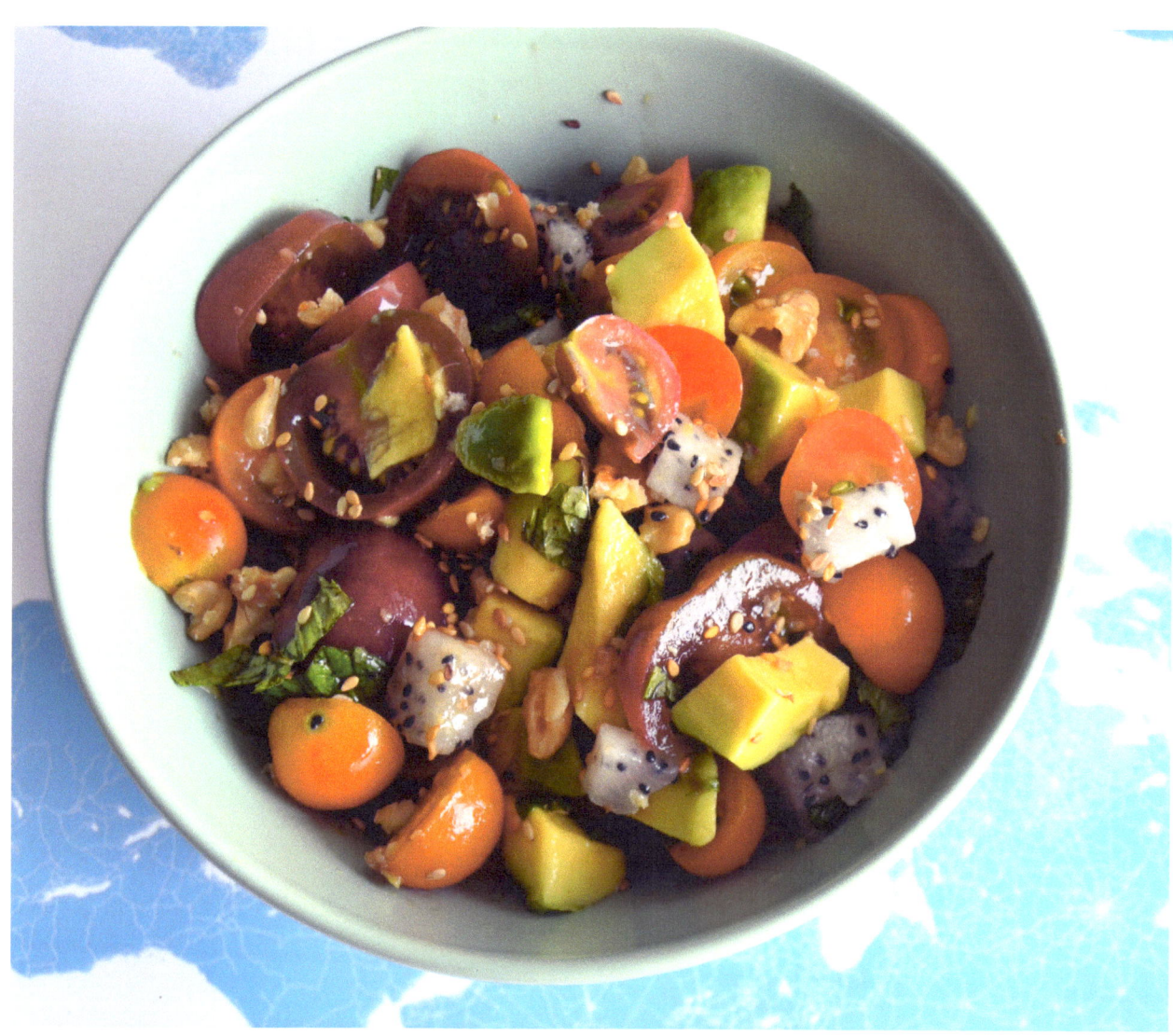

CAPRESE AVOCADO PITAYA SALAD

Time - 15 minutes
Serves - 2

Ingredients
100 g pitaya
50 ml pomegranate syrup
130 g cherry tomatoes
1 ripe avocado
1/4 cup fresh basil leaves
1 tbsp olive oil
1 tsp lemon juice
A handful raw walnuts
1 tbsp sesame seeds
1/4 tsp salt

1. Peel your pitaya and cut into cubes.

2. Cut the tomatoes in halves. Add the pitaya cubes, tomatoes, avocado, fresh basil into a large bowl.

3. Pour some olive oil, pomegeranate syrup and lemon juice. Then gently toss them until they are coated well.

4. Season generously with salt and pepper and toss just briefly.

5. Sprinkle some sesame and walnuts. Serve!

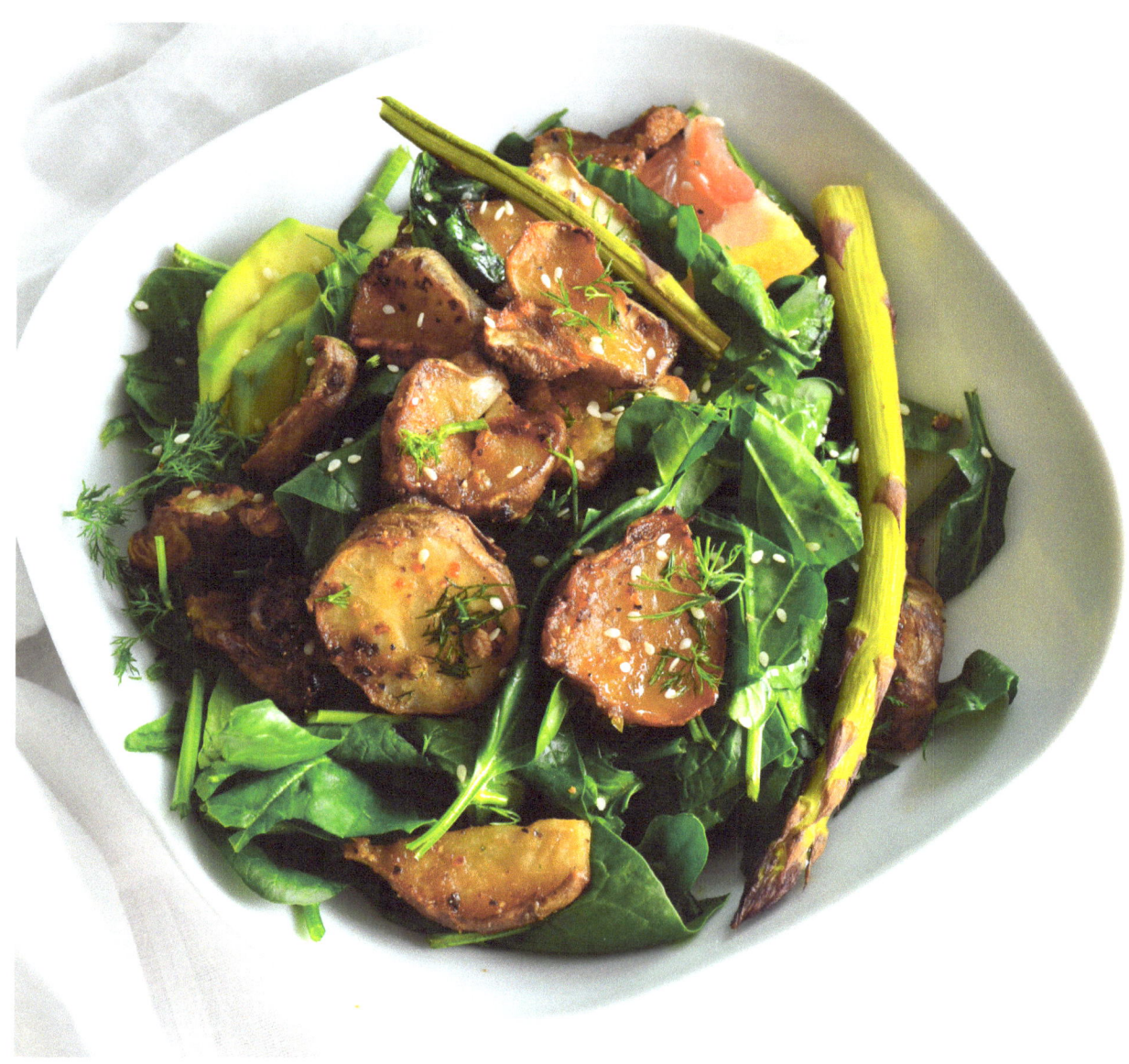

ROASTED SUNCHOKES WITH SPINACH AND ASPARAGUS

Time - 45 minutes
Serves - 3-4

Ingredients
400 g sunchokes
1 tbsp olive oil
1 tbsp tamari or soy sauce
1 tsp ground bay leaf
1 tsp thyme
1 tsp garlic powder
1 tbsp maple syrup
1/2 bunch asparagus
1 tsp ground mustard
Salt and pepper to taste
2 tbsp fresh dill
1 avocado sliced
Sesame seeds to serve

1. Wash and brush your sunchokes to clean. Slice them thinly.

2. Pre-heat oven to 200° C.
Mix olive oil, tamari, garlic powder, thyme, mustard, bay leaf, tamari, maple syrup, pepper and salt in a large bowl. Place sunchokes and asparagus in the bowl, toss with the sauce.

3. Transfer sunchokes and asparagus onto the baking tray lined parchment paper.

4. Roast for 25-30 minutes until golden.

5. Serve with chopped dill, spinach, avocado, and sesame seeds.

CAULIFLOWER AND ALMOND GRATIN WITH LEMON BALM PESTO

Time - 50 minutes
Serves - 4 as a side

1 large caulilower, cut in ½ then each ½ into 6-8 large wedges, keeping the stalk and any lighter inner leaves intact
50 g cassava (or brown rice flour, tapioca, arrowroot)
50 g vegan butter
500 ml almond milk
100 g almonds chopped
1 tsp dijon mustard
Salt and pepper to taste

A lighter relation to cauliflower, this is an easy-to-make, gluten-free dish of cauliflower mixed with mustard , delicate almond milk and topped with crunchy flaked almonds. It makes a good, midweek main eaten with brown rice or quinoa and sautéed cabbage or kale.

1. Preheat oven to 220° C.
2. Steam or boil the cauliflower for 4-5 minutes. Drain and put to one side, so any excess moisture evaporates of.
3. Meanwhile, melt the vegan butter in a pan. Add the flour and stir on a very low heat for 2 minutes. Remove from the heat, add 3-4 tablespoon of the almond milk and whisk together to make a thick smooth paste. Gradually add the rest of the milk, whisking all the time, until the sauce is smooth.
4. Return to the heat, add the cheese and gently heat for a few minutes, until the cheese has melted and the sauce thickened. Stir in the mustard and season to taste.
5. Put the cauliflower in a baking dish. Pour over the sauce and sprinkle over a little extra cheese. Bake for 15 minutes.
6. Sprinkle over the almonds and bake for a further 10-15 minutes or so, until the almonds are golden.

NORDIC RED CABBAGE SALAD

Time - 45 minutes
Serves - 4 as a side

1 red onion thinly sliced
1 tbsp balsamic
1/2 head red cabbage tough core and ribs are removed, leaves finely shredded
1 red apple cored and thinly sliced
1/4 cup dried cranberries or raisins
1/2 tsp allspice
3 juniper berries, bashed with the lat of your knife
1 bay leaf
1/4 tsp cinnamon
100 ml water

Many red cabbage recipes take a good couple of hours to cook. This Scandinavian-inspired recipe has lots of warm spicy flavour but takes less than half the time so it's quick enough for midweek cooking. Serve it alongside potatoes, tempeh or on the top of open face sandwiches.

1. Heat the balsamic in a large wide frying pan, wok or casserole, one with a lid (or you can cover the cabbage with a layer of foil instead).
2. Add the onion and cabbage and fry for 10 minutes on a low to medium heat, stirring now and then.
3. Add the juniper, all spice, bay leaf, cinnamon, water and cranberry. Season, cover and cook on a low heat for 20 minutes.
4. Add the apple and cook for a further 20 minutes, stirring now and then to stop it catching. Check the seasoning before serving.

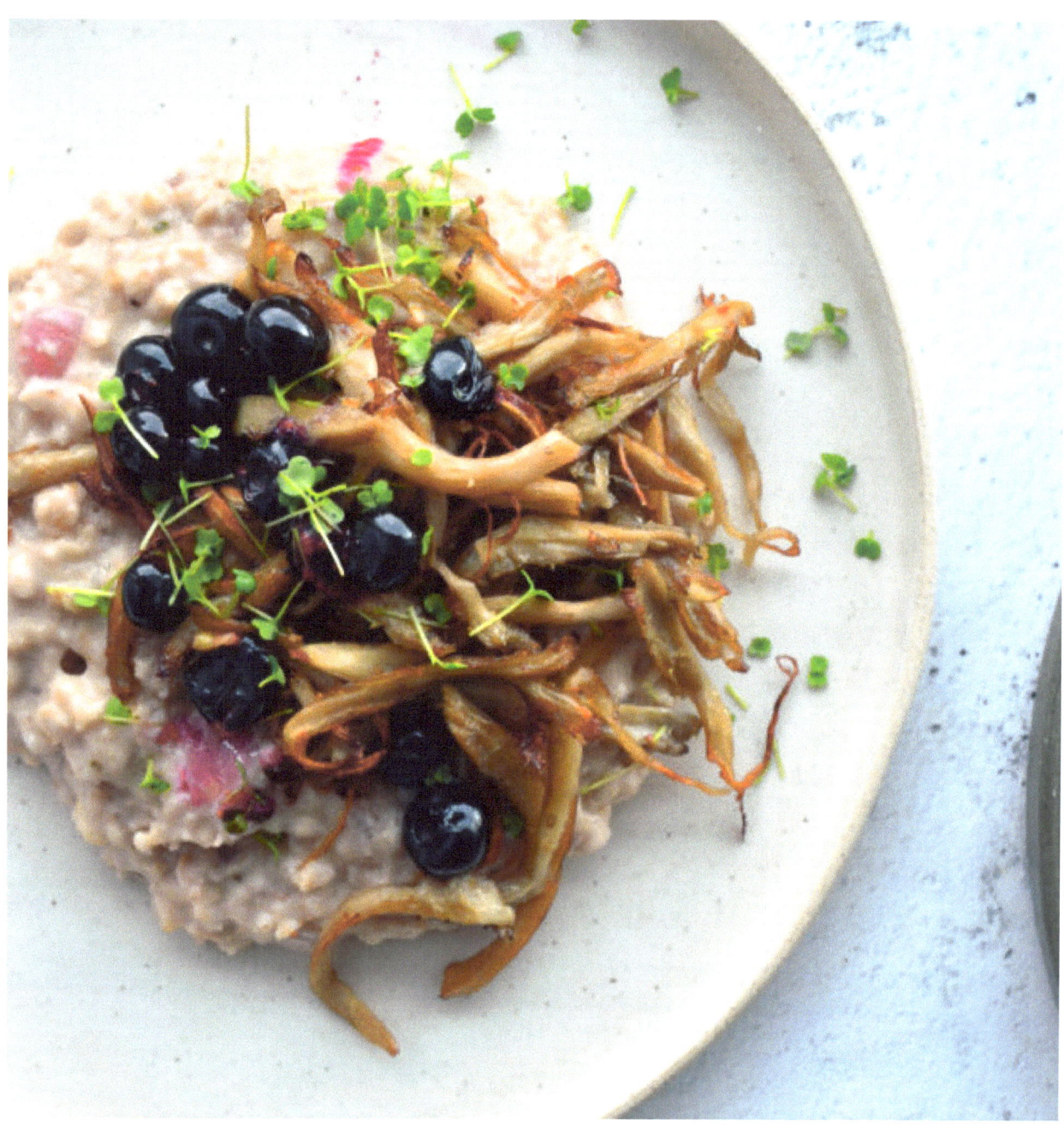

SAVORY PORRIDGE WITH MUSHROOM AND BERRIES

Time - 40 minutes
Serves - 2

Ingredients
130 g gluten free rolled oats
400 ml walnut milk
1 tbsp extra virgin olive oil
1 tsp salt
1 red onion chopped caramelized in the pan
1 tbsp dried rosemary
1 cup pulled oyster mushrooms (see below)
1 dl fresh blueberries or lingonberries
Plant based parmesan to serve

Pulled Oyster Mushrooms
400 g oyster mushrooms
1 tbsp tomato paste
1 tbsp olive oil
1/2 tsp chili pepper
1/2 tsp thyme
1 tsp salt
1 tsp garlic powder
1 tsp onion powder

1. Pour boiling water into the cup of dried rosemary until they are fully covered. Make sure to cover your rosemary with a visible level of water above them. This will ensure that rosemary absorbs the water well and it becomes very soft. Place a lid on top of the glass bowl to maintain the temperature. You can use fresh rosemary as well.
2. Place rolled oats in a pot. Pour the plant milk over the oats. Add the soften rosemary. Cook until oats absorb the milk and become creamy.
3. Add the caramelized onions into cooked oats. Stir well.
4. Add the salt and olive oil. Taste and adjust the flavour.
5. Divide between two plates.
6. Top with pulled oyster mushrooms.
7. Add some blueberries and micro greens. Serve immediately!

Pulled Oyster Mushrooms
1. Preheat oven to 200° C.
2. Clean mushrooms with a damp paper towel. (Do not wash the mushrooms) Using your hands, pull the mushrooms into thins strips.
3. Drizzle olive oil, add the rest of the ingredients.
4. Massage well with your hands. Toss around to evenly coat the mushrooms.
5. Transfer mushrooms in a baking tray lined parchment paper.
6. Bake at 200° C for 20-25 minutes or until mushrooms are a bit crispy and brown on the edges.
7. Serve with porridge, rice, potatoes or whatever you like.

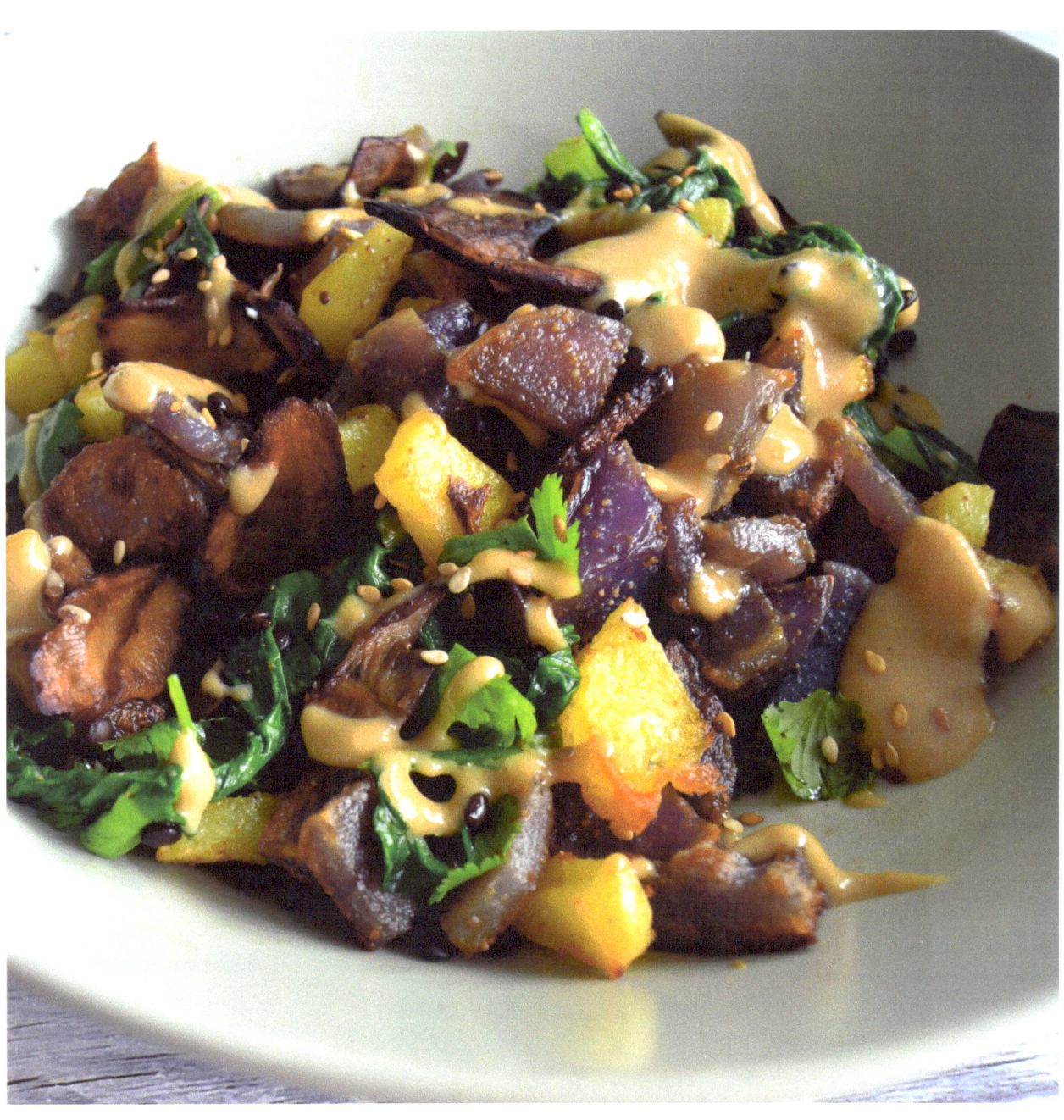

POTATO SALAD WITH CHARD, PORCINI, BELUGA AND GINGER TAHINI DRESSING

Time - 40 minutes
Serves - 2-3

Ingredients
70 g porcini mushrooms
2 tbsp grapeseed oil
2 tbsp shoyu
1 tsp garlic powder
2 tbsp fresh parsley
250 g purple potatoes
50 g yukon gold potatoes
70 g beluga lentils
6-7 leaves of swiss chard
1 tbsp sesame seeds
1 tsp sea salt

Dressing
4-5 tbsp tahini
1 tbsp grated fresh ginger
2 tbsp tamari
2 tbsp grape molasses
1 tsp habanero
2 tbsp spring water

1. Brush, wash and drain your mushrooms, if you will use dried mushrooms, then soak them in warm water at least 15 minutes and strain. Set aside.

2. In a large skillet, heat grapeseed oil, add shoyu and garlic powder. Transfer the mushrooms to the skillet, cook until golden.
3. Bake potatoes at 220° C for about 25-30 minutes in the oven or until golden.

4. In a pan, heat a bit olive oil in a large pan, add swiss chards, sprinkle salt. Saute on high heat for 1-2 minutes. Set aside.

5. Wash and strain beluga lentils. Cover with water and cook for 20 minutes or until tender.

6. Place swiss chards into a bowl, add the roasted potatoes, mushrooms and lentils. Sprinkle some parsley.

7. Place all sauce ingredients into a blender, mix until smooth. Use more or less water to achieve desired consistency.

8. Pour mixture over the bowl. Sprinkle sesame seeds. Serve. Decorate with sesame seeds and cilantro. Serve warm.

MAINS

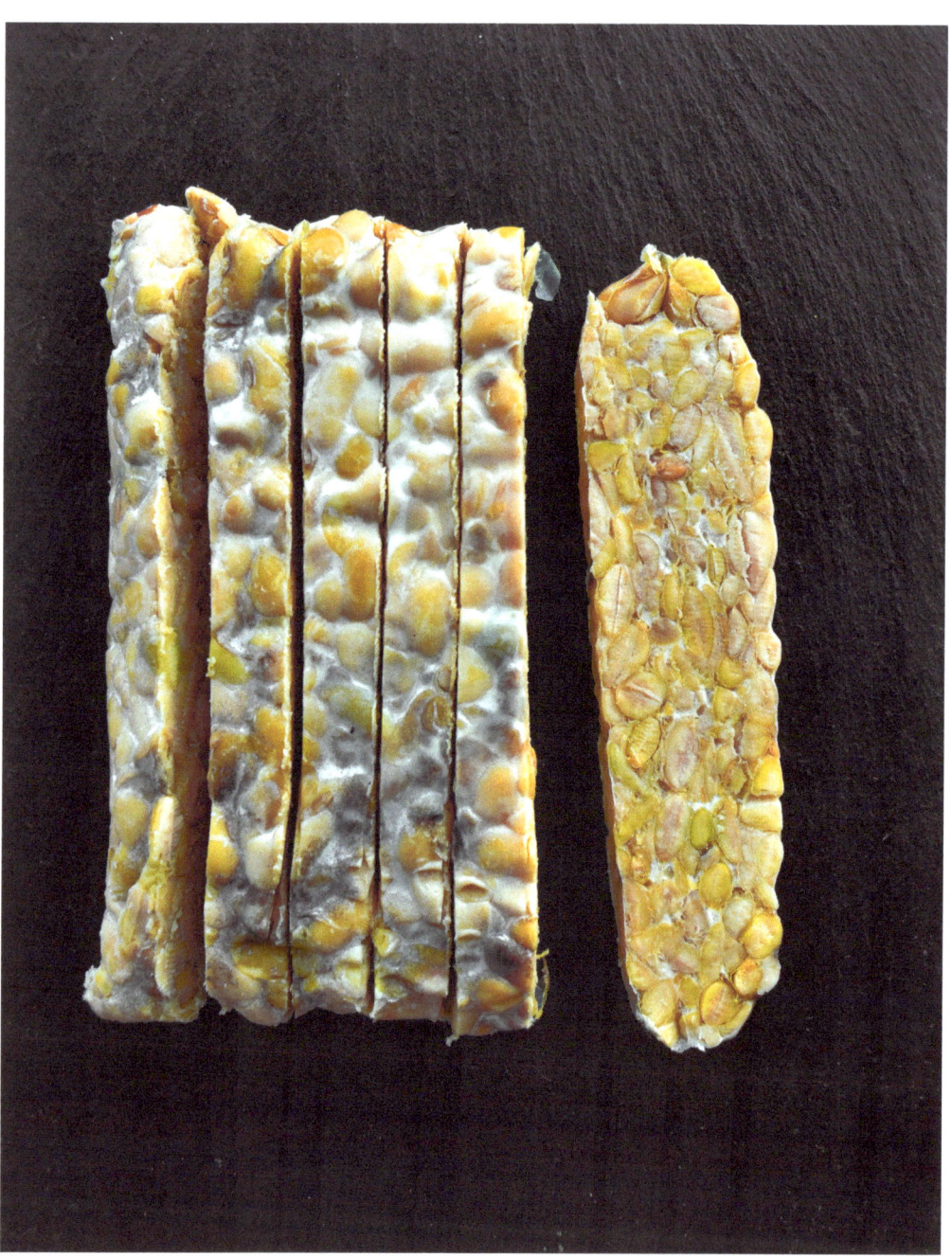

MAKING TEMPEH FROM SCRATCH

Time - 3-4 days
Serves - 3-4

Ingredients
1 cup dry chickpeas or soy beans
1 tbsp white vinegar
1 tsp tempeh starter

1. Place the chickpeas in a large bowl, cover with clean water soak for 8 hours or overnight.
2. The next day, drain and rinse the chickpeas. Transfer to a large cooking pot, cover with water (about 2-inch higher than the chickpeas). Bring to a boil and let simmer for 1 hour. Depending on the size of your chickpeas it might take up to 1 and 1/2 hour. They must be soft but not mushy. If some foam forms on the surface during cooking, remove it with a spoon to prevent any spillover.
3. Once the chickpeas are cooked, drain them and leave them in the strainer for 30 minutes. After that, pat them dry using a paper towel to make sure they are mostly dry on the outside. Transfer to a large clean bowl. Add the white vinegar and stir to coat. Add the tempeh starter and mix well using a spoon until uniformly distributed. Using a metal skewer, or chopstick, prick some holes (at about 2-inch intervals) in a clean freezer bag. This step is important to create good air circulation and allow the mold to grow.
4. Transfer the chickpeas to the freezer bag and form a rectangle of about 5×8 inches with a thickness of about 1-inch. Place the bag of chickpeas on a baking sheet and put in an oven with the light on for about 14 hours. I set the temperature of my oven to 86°F and let the door very slightly opened because I can't just let the light on.
5. After 14 hours, some white mold (not a lot) should have appeared on the chickpeas. You might also see some condensation inside the plastic bag, this is normal. It's time to remove the baking sheet from the oven and let it ferment for another 24-36H in a dark and warm place. I recommend covering the chickpea bag with a clean towel to make sure it's not under direct sunlight.
6. Your tempeh is ready when it is fully covered with white mold and forms a solid cake, which usually happens at the 48-hour mark. It can be quicker if the temperature in your house is high.

Raw tempeh will keep for up to a week in the refrigerator. If you want to freeze it: steam the tempeh for 25 minutes, let cool completely and wrap in plastic film before freezing.

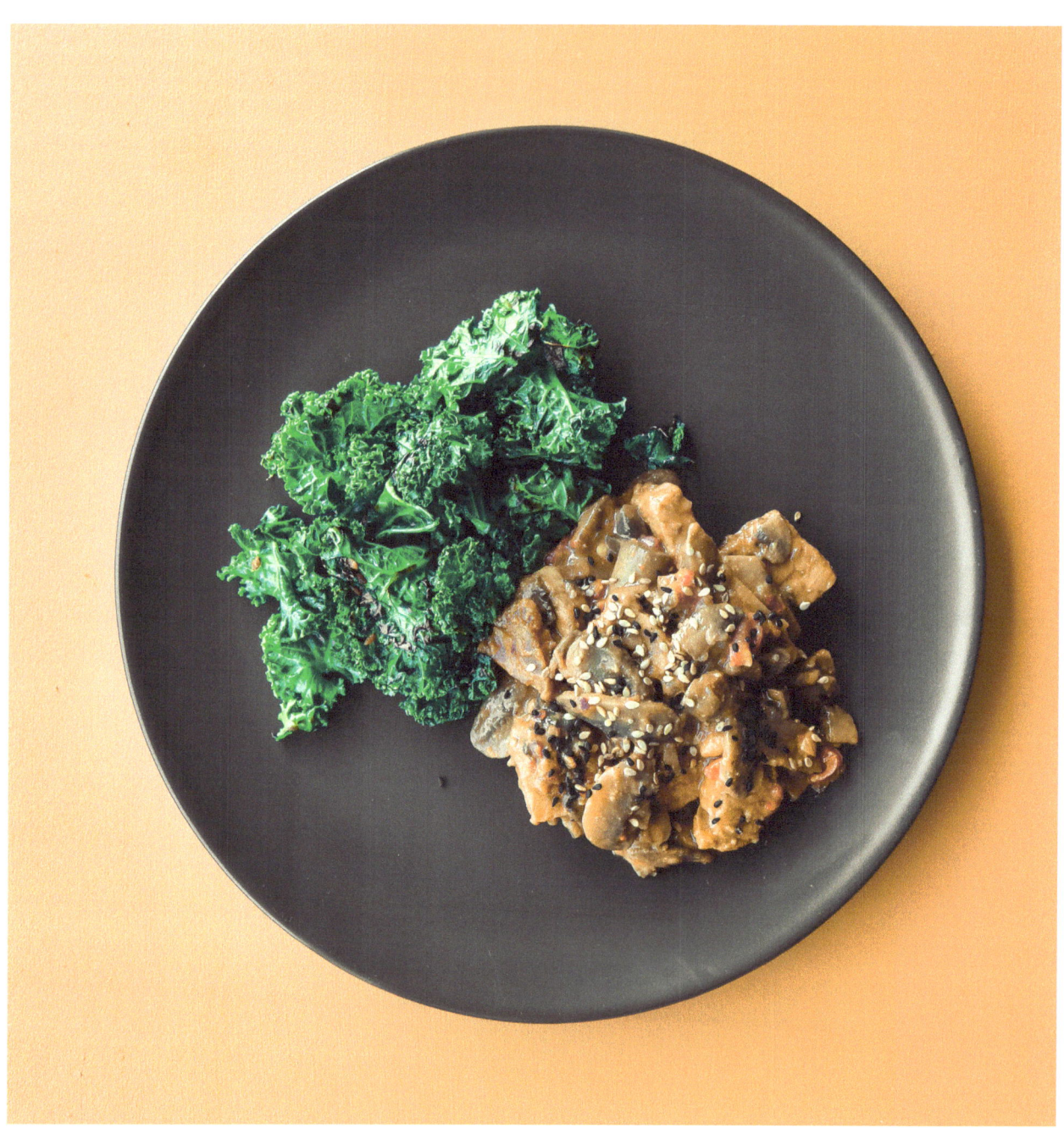

TEMPEH WITH MUSHROOM COCONUT SAUCE & KALE

Time - 1 hour
Serves - 2-3

Tempeh
250 g tempeh
2 tbsp tamari
1 tbsp maple syrup
2 cups kale

Mushroom Coconut Sauce
1 shallot chopped finely
3 garlic cloves minced
1 tbsp olive oil
350 g mushrooms sliced
1 tbsp tamari
1/4 cup coconut cream
1/2 cup water
1/8 tsp salt
1/8 tsp blackpepper
1/2 tsp chili
1 tsp tapioca if needed
Fresh parsley chopped

1. Cut the tempeh into 1-inch cubes and place them in a deep plate or baking dish. In a small bowl, prepare the marinade by combining the tamari sauce, maple syrup, and garlic. Pour the marinade over the tempeh and stir to coat. Let the tempeh marinade for at least 30 minutes, or overnight in the refrigerator.
2. Once tempeh has marinated, heat a tablespoon of oil in a non-stick skillet. Add the tempeh with the marinade and cook for about 5 minutes, or until the tempeh has absorbs the marinade and starts to brown. Remove from heat and set aside.
3. To make mushroom sauce, heat a tablespoon of oil in a large non-stick skillet over medium heat. Once hot, add the onion and garlic and fry until golden brown. Next, add the sliced mushrooms and cook for 5-7 minutes, or until mushrooms are cooked and start to brown.
4. Deglaze the skillet with the tamari sauce. Add the maple syrup, ground black pepper, salt, coconut cream, and water. Stir to combine and cook for another 5 minutes. If you want to thicken the sauce, add a teaspoon tapioca.
5. Add the sautéed tempeh to the skillet and cook for another 5 minutes. Top with fresh chopped parsley.
Tempeh and the sauce will keep for up to 3 days in the refrigerator.
6. Wash and dry your kale, place in a hot pan, drizzle little bit olive oil and saute on high heat for 2-3 minutes. Once done, remove from the heat. Serve with your tempeh.

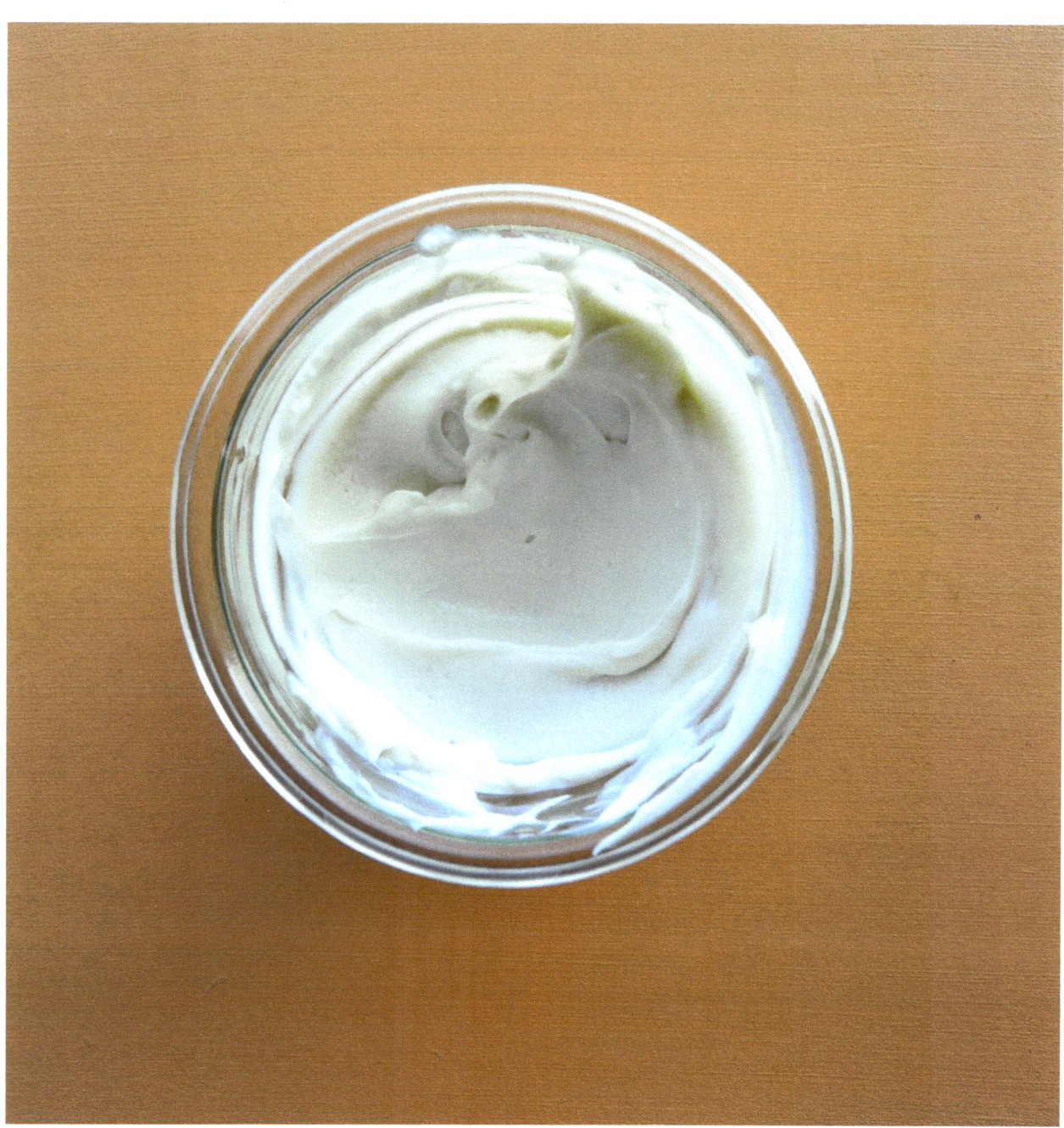

OAT COCONUT YOGURT

Time - 15 minutes prep + 14 hrs fermentation
Serves - 3-4

Ingredients
400 ml oat milk
60 g young coconut meat
1 acidophilus probiotic capsule
1 tbsp tapioca or cassava flour
1 tbsp maple
1/4 tsp salt

1. Place young coconut meat in the blender.
2. Add the oat milk, maple, salt and tapioca or cassava. Blend until smooth.
3. Transfer mixture in a saucepan. Cook on medium heat for 4-5 minutes until warm but not boiling.
4. Remove from the heat and let it cool.
5. When it is warm, add the acidophilus capsule and stir well.
6. Transfer to a mason jar, close the lid with a clean cheesecloth.
7. Let it ferment at 36° C in the dehydrator for 14 hours.
8. It should be tangy and fresh at the end. Taste it and transfer to your fridge.
9. It will become thicken in the fridge after 4-5 hours sitting. It can be kept up to a week.

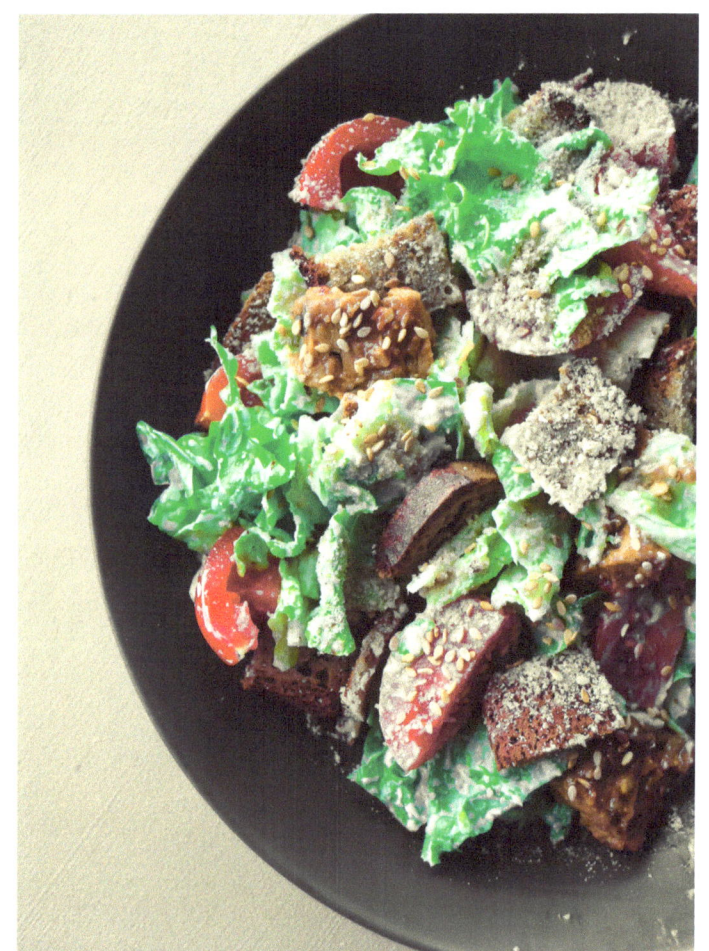
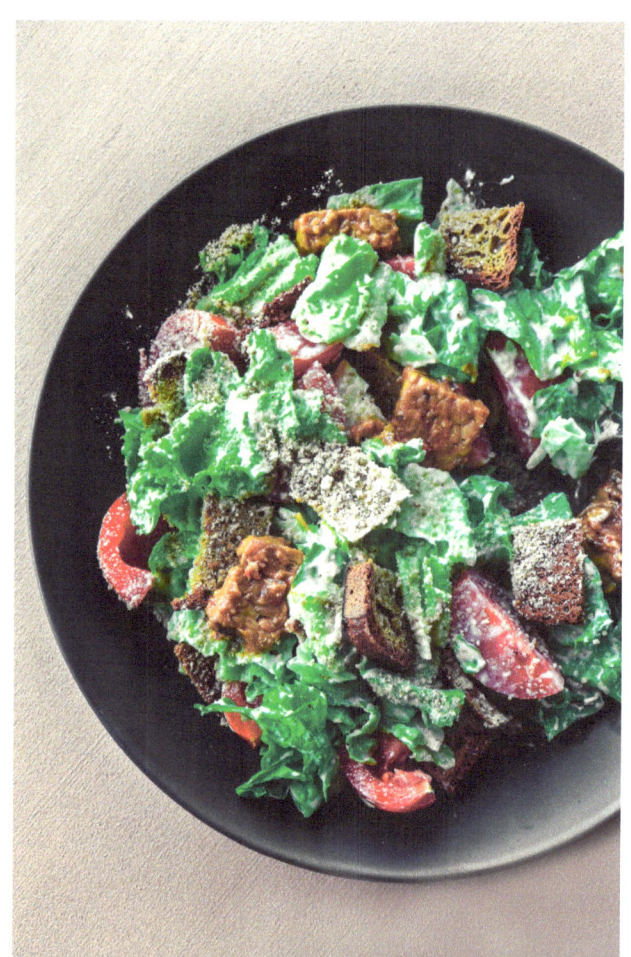

CREAMY CEASAR SALAD WITH TEMPEH

Time - 30 minutes
Serves - 2

Ingredients
1 cup oat coconut yogurt (check previous page)
5-6 slices of old day bread
2 tbsp olive oil
2 cups cherry tomatoes halved
1-2 tbsp lemon juice
1 tsp dijon mustard
1 large romanie lettuce
2 garlic cloves minced
170 g grilled tempeh (check "tempeh making from scratch" recipe or use store-bought one.)
1/4 cup nut parmesan or fermented vegan cheese (find the recipe in the bite sizes chapter)
Salt and pepper to taste

1. Preheat oven to 200° C. Add the old bread cubes to a silicone mat on a baking sheet or a baking sheet prepared with parchment paper or foil.

2. Drizzle the olive oil over the cubes, and sprinkle with salt and pepper. Toss gently with hands to coat. Bake for 5 minutes. Remove from oven and set aside to cool.

3. Place the yogurt in a bowl, add the minced garlic, mustard and a little bit lemon juice. Stir together.

4. In a large mixing bowl, add the chopped lettuce. Drizzle a good amount of yogurt lettuce and toss to combine.

5. Add in toasted bread, halved tomatoes, coconut bacon (find the recipe in the bite sizes chapter) or grilled tempeh and the vegan parmesan cheese. Toss until combined. Adjust the salt and pepper.

6. If you will use the grilled tempeh, first marinate in the 1 tbsp maple and 2 tbsp tamari for at least one hour, then grill or fry in the pan. Cut into cubes and add to your salad.

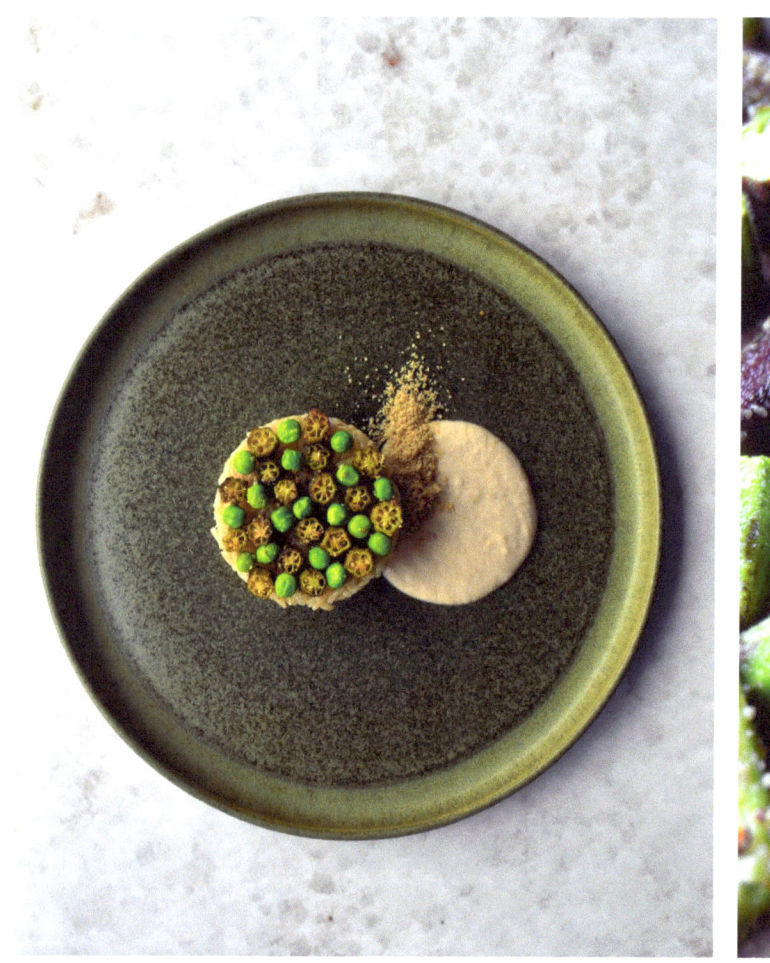
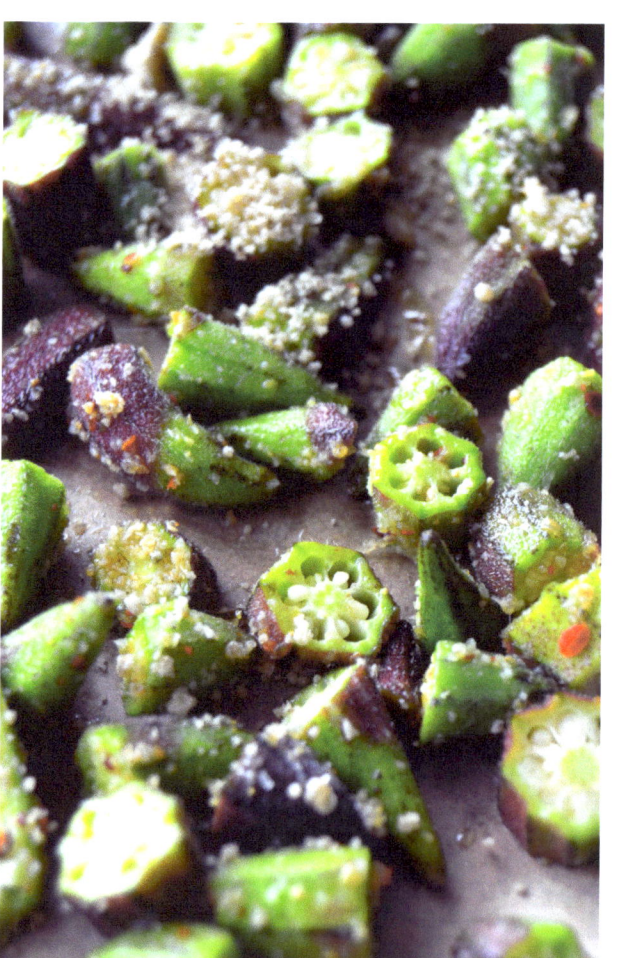

BROWN RICE AND OKRA WITH PEAR CREAM

Time - 10 min prep + 25 min baking
Serves - 2

Ingredients
200 g brown rice
2 cups filtered water
1 cup okra
1 cup green peas
1 tbsp olive oil
1 tsp garlic powder
1/2 tsp salt

Pear Cream
1 ripe pear
1 red onion
1 garlic cloves
65 g oat crème fraiche
1/2 tsp salt

1. Wash the brown rice and in a pot cover with water, let it sit for 1 hour while you are preparing other components.
2. Wash the okra under running water, then dry throughly, then remove caps and slice the okra into 1/3" thick round pieces. Place in a bowl, add the olive oil, salt and garlic powder. Give it a good toss. Then transfer to a baking tray lined parchment paper. Preheat oven to 200° C and bake for 10-12 minutes both side of the okra rounds. Check it. If the pieces are still soggy, put them back for an additional 5-10 minutes. Be sure to move the pieces around frequently so the okra browns on all sides. The okra will be a dark green-brown colour, and will smell a bit nutty when it's cooked through. The edges should be a bit crisp and the middle should be tender. The longer you leave the okra in the oven, the smaller and darker they will get so be careful not to overcook them.
3. In a parge pan, with little olive oil fry the fresh or defrosted peas on medium-high heat until they are bright green and soft enough. Sprinkle some salt and garlic powder. Set aside.

MAINS

4. Chop your onion, garlic and pear, place in a large pan. Drizzle a little bit olive oil and cook on mediim heat until they are soften, add 1 tbsp water if you need. Once they are soften, add the oat crème fraiche and salt. Continue to cook for 1-2 minutes. Then transfer mixture into a blender. Blend until you get smooth cream. Then transfer back to the pot. Cook on medium heat until the sauce becomes thick enough. Set aside.

5. Drain your brown rice and rinse then add 2 cups filltered water and bring to boil. Reduce heat and simmer covered for 15 minutes until becomes tender. Let the rice rest, off the heat, for 10 minutes. Fluff, season as desired, and serve.

6. Using a round pastry cutter, shape your rice in the middle of the plate.

7. Cover the top of the rice by lining up the peas and okra in order.

8. Pour 2 tbsp of pear sauce right next to the rice. Sprinkle some rawmesan if desired. Serve immediately.

SWEDISH POTATO DUMPLINGS

Time - 1 hour
Serves - 3-4 person

Ingredients
400 g potatos peeled and cut into quarters
65 g quinoa flour plus extra for dusting
Salt and pepper to taste

Sauce
1 large onion
2 garlic cloves
1 tbsp vegetable broth
150 g chopped mushrooms, tofu or pea mince
1 tsp salt
1/2 tsp fresh ground black pepper

1. Fresh lingonberries or lingonberry jam.
2. Sautéd dinosaur kale and chanterelles.
3. Chop the onion and garlic, in a large pan fry with little olive oil until soften. Then add the chopped mushrooms or tofu or pea mince, continue to cook until the mixture gets golden brown. Transfer to a bowl and set aside.
4. Place the potatos into a pan of boiling water and simmer for about 20 minutes until cooked.
5. Drain the potatos, give them a shake to remove as much of the cooking water as possible, and leave in the sieve to dry and cool.
6. Once dry place in a bowl and chop then mash until smooth, or pass through a potato ricer.
7. Season then add the quinoa flour and work it in using your hands.   Add as much flour as you need to make a smooth dough that stick together.
8. Shape the dough into a log with floured hands and cut in small pieces. Make 6 little pocket in each piece and fill with 2 tablespoon of the filling. Close and shape to a ball. Make sure the filling is covered everywhere.
9. Place the dumplings in a pan with little veg stock and fry until they get a golden crispy crust.
10. Serve the crispy dumplings with berries, kale and oat cream.

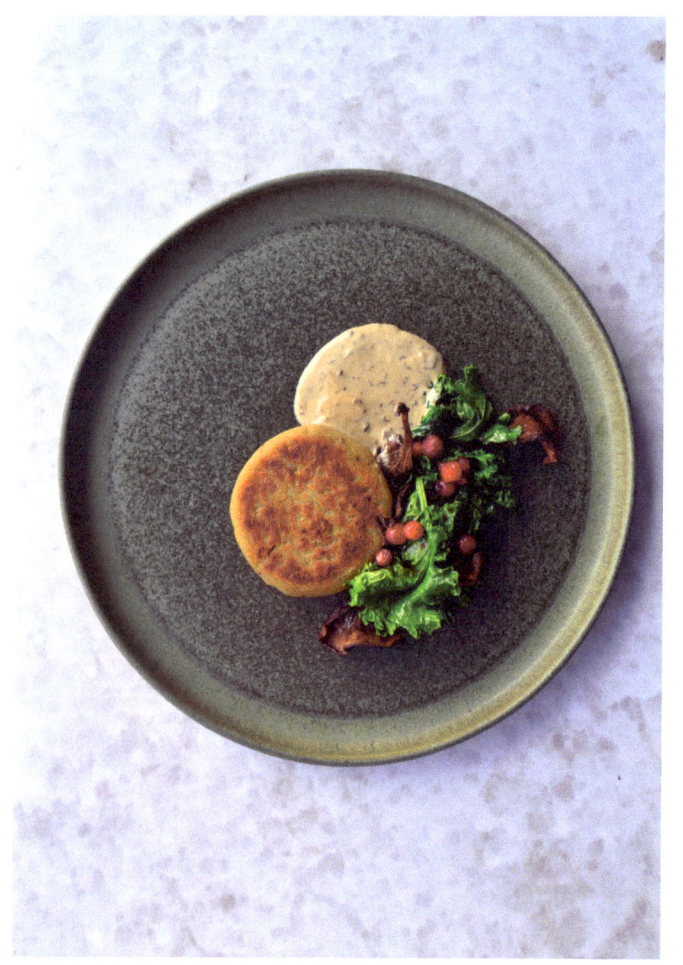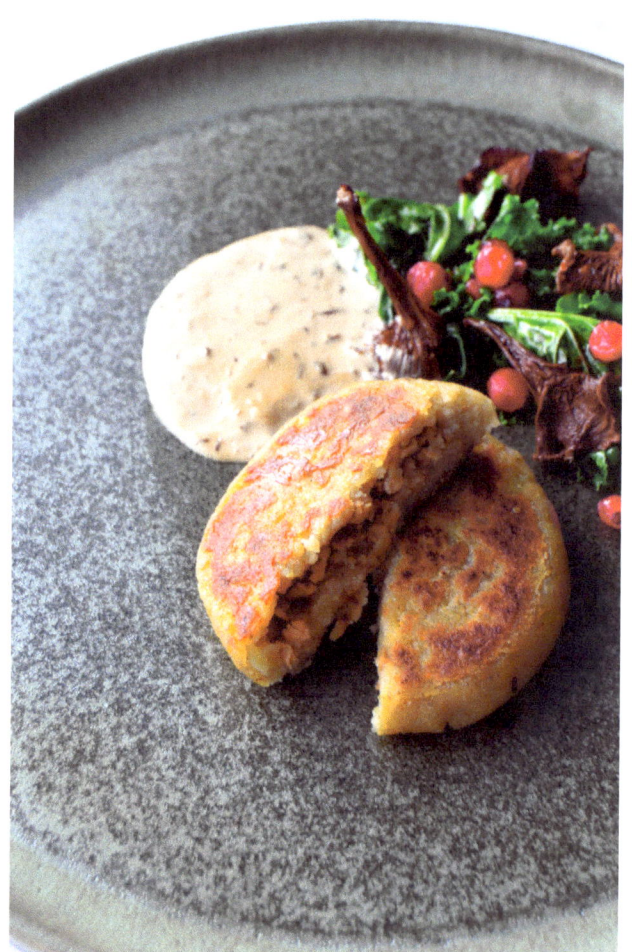

Potato dumplings continued

Sautéd Kale and Chantarelles

¼ cup extra-virgin olive oil
3 cloves garlic, peeled and sliced
1 large bunch kale, stemmed, with leaves coarsely chopped
150 g chanterelles
1/2 cup vegetable stock, white wine or water
Sea salt, freshly ground black pepper and red-pepper flakes to taste
2 tablespoons orange juice

To sauté kale leaves, heat little olive oil in a large sauté pan set over medium-high heat until it shimmers.
Add garlic, and cook until soft. Add the mushrooms to the pan, turn the heat to high and add the stock. Cook until golden brown. Then add the kale leaves and use a spoon to toss the greens in the oil and stock, then cover and cook for approximately 5 to 7 minutes, until it is soft and wilted, but still quite green.
Remove cover and continue to cook, stirring occasionally until all the liquid has evaporated, another 1 to 2 minutes. Season to taste with salt and peppers, add orange juice and toss to combine.

Oat chanterelle Cream

Ingredients:
1 package oatly imat
1 tbsp chanterelle powder
1 tbsp tamari

Preheat a large non stick pan.
Add the oat cream, chanterelle powder and tamari. Whisk well.
Cook until thicken. Serve with your dumplings.

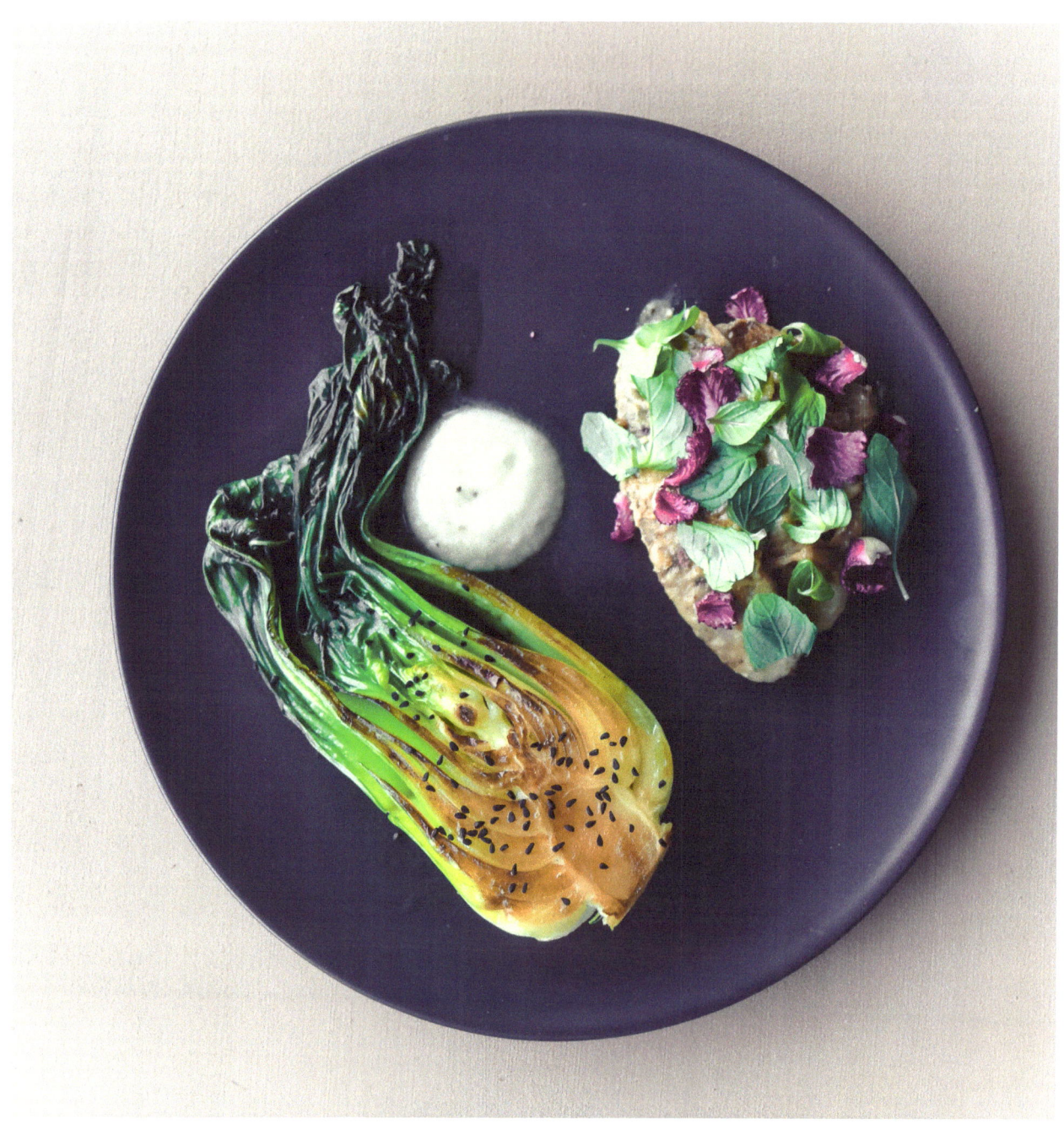

TEMPEH SATAY WITH SPICY HAZELNUT-GINGER SAUCE

Tempeh

350 g tempeh
4 tbsp olive oil
1/4 cup water
1/4 cup tamari
1 tbsp grape molasses
1 tsp chili
Lemon wedges to serve
Fresh parsley to serve
Chili to serve
Sesame to serve
Grilled bok choy to serve

Spicy Hazelnut-Ginger Sauce

1/2 cup smooth hazelnut butter
2 tbsp tamari
1/4 cup lemon juice
1/2 cup water to thin
1 tbsp freshly greated ginger
2 garlic cloves minced
1/2 tsp chili

1. Thinly slice your tempeh cut into strips.
2. Heat a pan on medium heat. Add the olive oil and tempeh strips.
3. After 1-2 minutes, using another heavy pan, weight down and press the tempeh. After 2 minutes, add the water, tamari, grape molasses and chili.
4. Continue cooking and pressing for 2-3 minutes, then flip the tempeh over.
5. When the tempeh strips are tender and absorbed all the water content, remove from the heat. Let cool for 5-10 minutes.
6. Place all spicy hazelnut-ginger sauce ingredients in a blender, blend until smooth. Transfer sauce in a airtight container.
7. Place tempeh strips in the hazelnut-ginger sauce. Let lt marinate for at least 2 hour. The longer you marinate, the more flavour you will have.
8. Once marinated, transfer marinated tempeh strips on a baking sheet, then brush them with the rest of hazelnut-ginger sauce. Keep some sauce aside to drizzle over the tempeh strips to serve if desired.
9. Bake at preheated 175° C for about 20-25 minutes or until lightly browned.
10. Serve with lemon wedges, grilled bok choi, chili slices or flakes and parsley. Sprinkle some sesame on top. Enjoy.

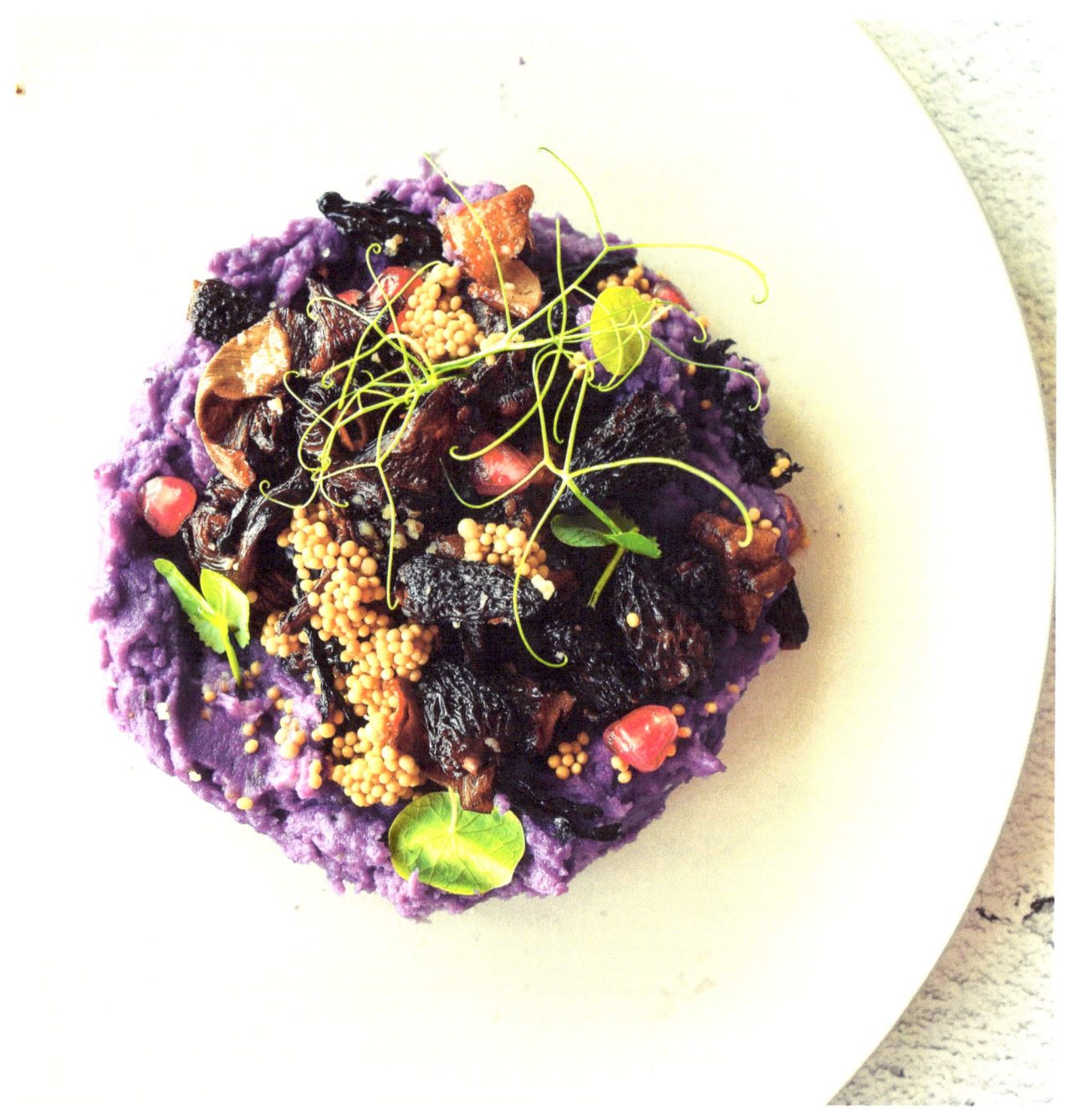

MASHED PURPLE POTATO WITH MIXED MUSHROOMS

Time - 40 minutes
Serves - 3-4 person

Ingredients for the mashed potatoes
400 g purple potato
4-5 garlic cloves
1 tsp salt
2-3 tbsp olive oil
4-5 tbsp almond milk

For the mushrooms
60 g. dried mushroom mix (morel, porcini, black trumpet, chantarelle)
1 tbsp olive oil
1/2 tsp salt

For the garnish
Pickled mustard seeds
Pomegranate seeds
Sprouted peas
Nasturtium leaves

1. Bring a pot of salted water to a boil. Add potatoes and cook until tender but still firm, about 15 minutes; drain and peel.
2. Transfer to a food processor. Add garlic cloves, salt, almond milk and olive oil. Mix until smooth and creamy.
3. Divide puree between the plates.
4. To make mushrooms, place dried mushrooms in a bowl, cover with warm water for 10 minutes. Strain and drain the mushrooms.
5. Heat a large pan with olive oil, add the mushrooms, cook until tender and crispy.
6. To assemble, add mushrooms on the top of mashed purple potatoes.
7. Add some pomegranate seeds, pickled mustard seeds using a teaspoon, sprouted peas and nasturtium leaves.
8. Serve warm. Enjoy!

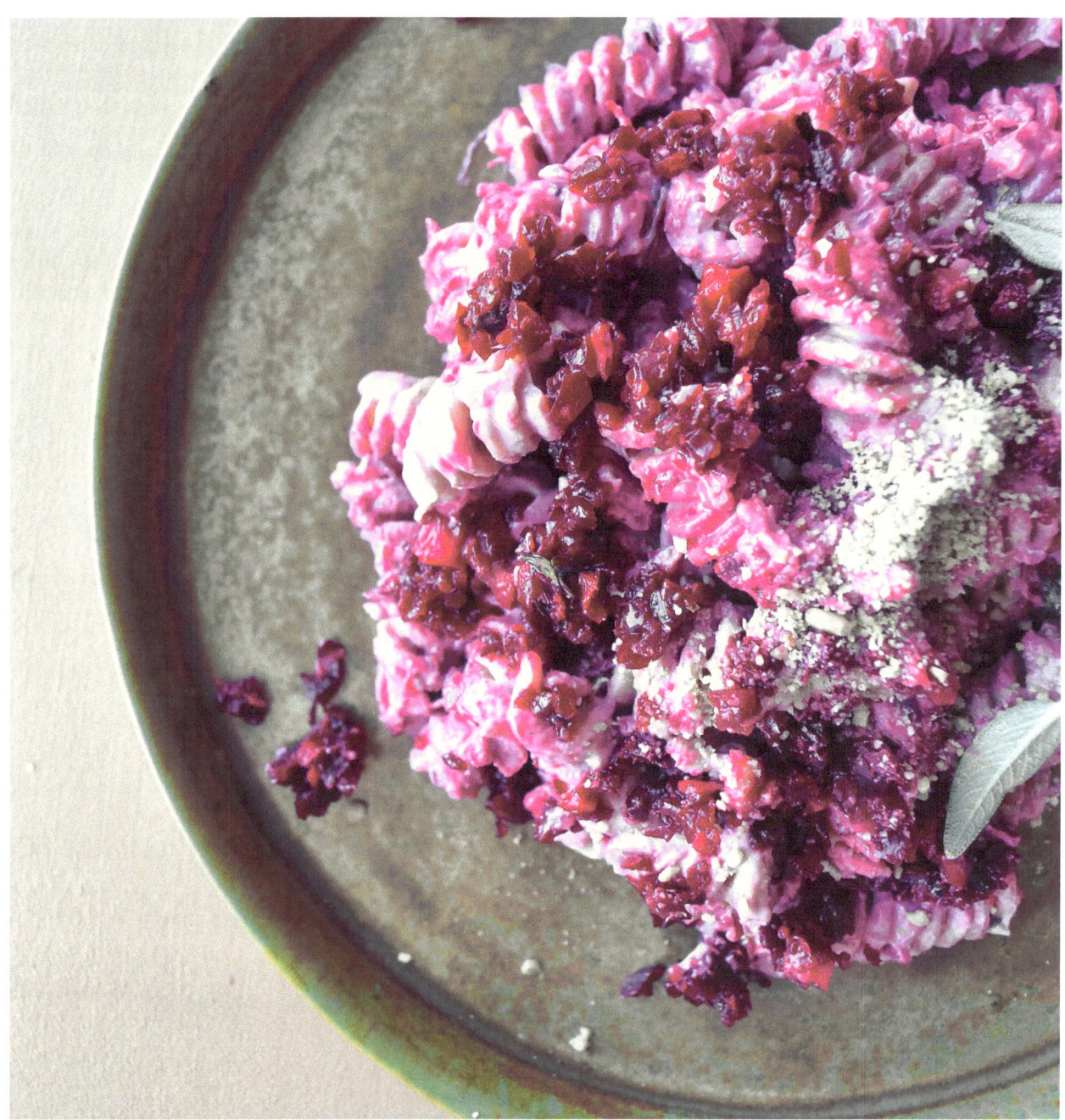

PASTA WITH CAULIFLOWER ALFREDO AND CRANBERRY PESTO

Time - 30 min
Serves - 2-3 person

Ingredients
250 g gf pasta of your choice
300 g cauliflower florets
1 cup cauliflower stock
Juice of 2 whole lemon
1/2 cup sunflower seed or almond flour
2 garlic cloves freshly grated
1 tsp salt
Nut parmesan to serve (optional)
Fresh sage leaves to serve (optional)

Beet Cranberry Pesto
175 g cooked beetroots
1/4 cup beetroot vegetable broth
5 tbsp plant milk
1 tbsp balsamic vinegar
1 medium red onion chopped
1 garlic cloves minced
1/4 bunch fresh parsley chopped
1/4 cup roasted pecan nuts or almonds
2 tbsp dried cranberries
Salt as needed

1. Wash and drain your cauliflower, place in a deep pot, cover with the water. Bring to boil until soften.
2. Once soften, strain and keep 1 cup water from the cooked cauliflower.
3. Place the cauliflower in a high speed blender. Add the cauliflower water, lemon juice, black pepper and salt. Process until smooth. Transfer cauliflower sauce in the pot, cook on medium heat until thick enough. Then add the sunflower seed flour, and stir well.
4. Cook your pasta according to package instructions. Once cooked strain and transfer back to the pot, toss with cauliflower sauce.
5. Place all the beet cranberry pesto ingredients in a food processor, blend until you get rice like texture. Transfer to a bowl. Top on the pasta. Serve with nut parmesan.

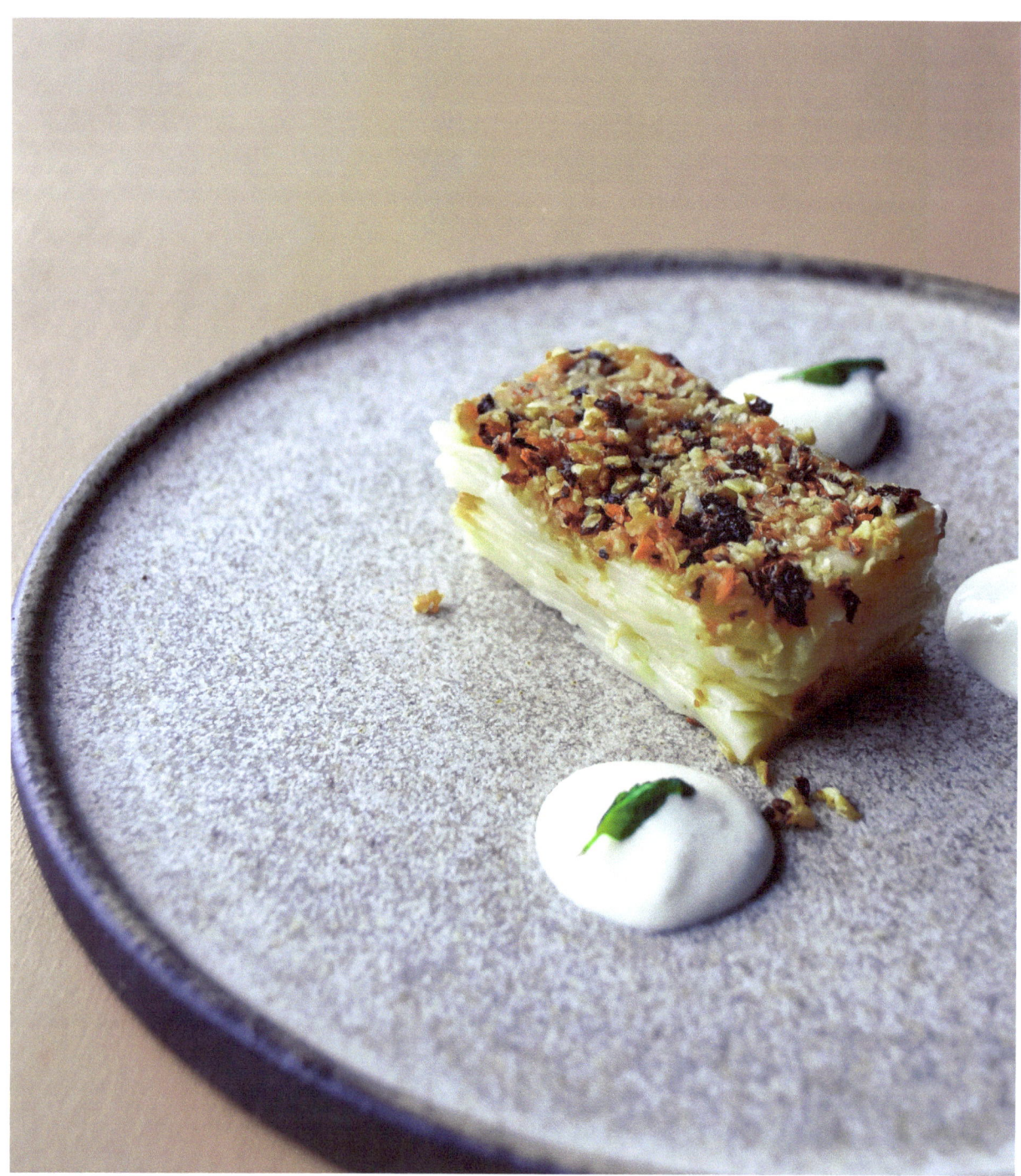

CELERIAC PAVE WITH CREAM AND CRUMB

Time - 2 hours
Serves - 4 person

Ingredients
700 g celeriac
1/4 cup olive oil
Salt to season
Vegan yogurt or cream cheese to serve

Celeriac crumb
1 large head celeriac
2 tbsp olive oil
1 tsp seaweed powder
Salt and pepper to taste
1 tbsp toasted sesame seeds
3 tbsp breadcrumbs

1. Preheat the oven to 180° C.
2. Peel the celeriac and slice on a mandoline as thin as possible.
3. Line a loaf pan with parchment and place down a layer of the celeriac slices, then brush with olive oil. Repeat this layering until all the celeriac has been used.
4. Cover the loaf pan with a lid or foil and bake for 1 hour 20 minutes or so, until the celeriac is tender. Allow to cool. Cut a sheet of parchment to lay on top of the terrine in the loaf pan and top with a heavy weight so that the terrine will compact and become stable for slicing.
5. Refrigerate overnight with the weight on top.
6. Remove the weights from the Celeriac Pavé, unmould and trim the edges if you prefer. Slice lengthwise into pieces. Place the pieces onto a parchment-lined baking sheet, brush some olive oil and warm gently in the oven for about 20 minutes.
7. Remove from the oven and top with a generous layer of celeriac crumb. Transfer to plates and top with dollops of vegan yogurt or cream cheese if desired.
8. To make celeriac crumb, place the celeriac in the food processor, process until rice-like texture. Transfer to a bowl, add the rest of the ingredients, toss well together.
9. Line baking tray with parchment paper, place the celeriac crumb, spread evenly.
10. Bake at 180° C for 20-25 minutes or until dry and crispy enough. Serve on the top of your pave.

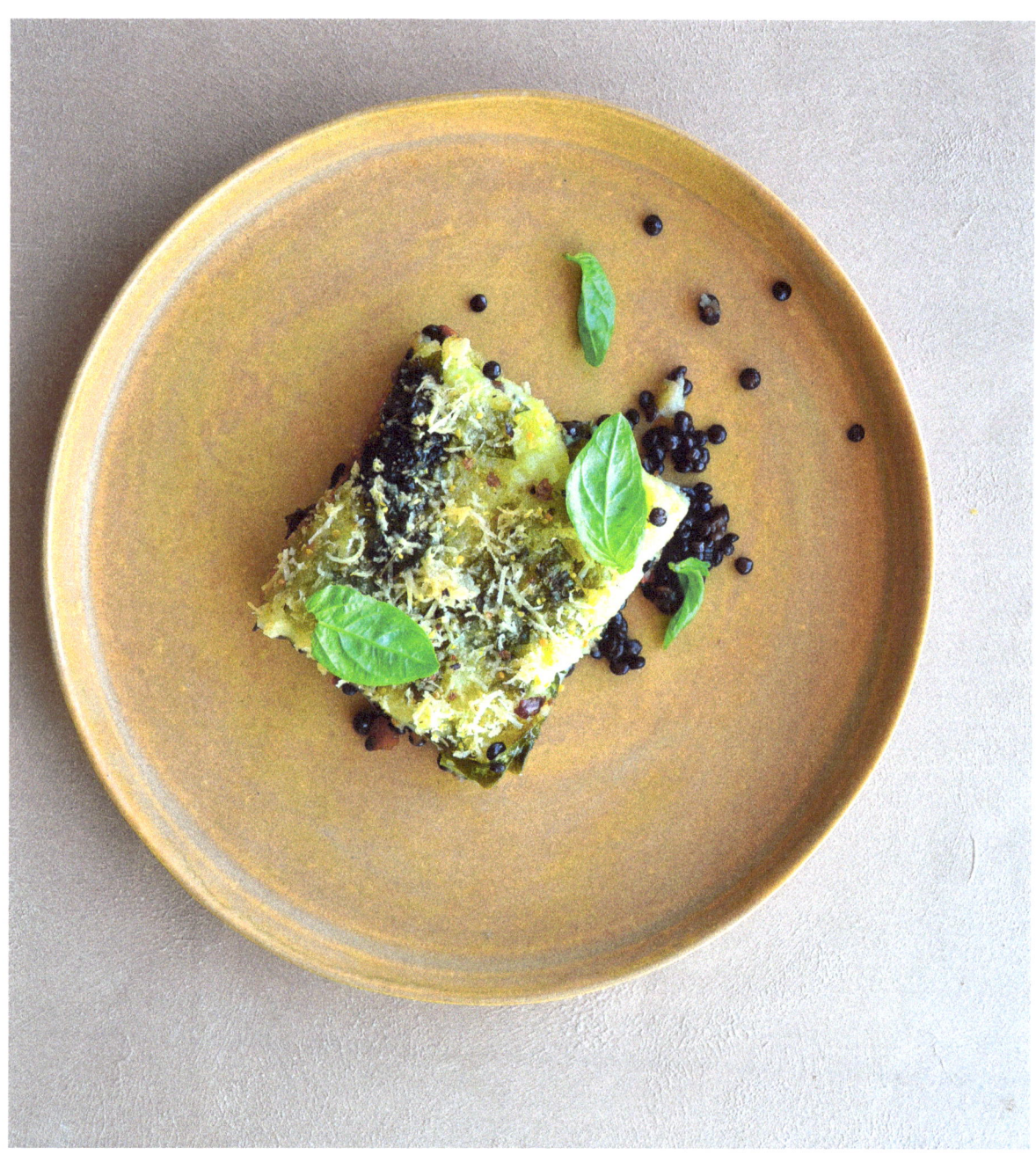

SHEPHERD'S PIE WITH BELUGA

Time - 1 hour
Serves - 4-6 person

Ingredients

700 g yukon gold potatoes
300 g celeriac
100 ml plant based milk
2-4 tbsp olive oil
1/2 tsp salt
Blackpepper to taste
Fresh parsley or basil chopped
Lemon wedges to serve

Filling

2 tbsp olive oil
150 g beluga lentils
1 tbsp soy sauce or tamari
2 carrots diced
2 sticks celery diced
1 large onion chopped
1/2 tsp salt
1/4 tsp blackpepper

1. Slice the potatoes in half, place in a large pot and fill with water until they're just covered. Bring to a low boil on medium high heat, then generously salt, cover and cook for 20-30 minutes or until they slide off a knife very easily. Peel your celeriac and repeat the process for it, just cook for 10-15 minutes or until soften.

2. Once cooked, drain, peel the potatoes, then transfer to a mixing bowl along with the celeriac. Use a masher or fork to mash until smooth (you can also shred them.) Add some olive oil, plant milk and season with salt and pepper. Loosely cover and set aside.

3. Preheat oven to 220° C and lightly grease a large square baking dish.

4. Cook the beluga lentils according the instructions on the package. Do not overcook, they should be tender as we will cook them in the oven.

5. In a large pan over medium heat, sauté the onions, carrots, celery and garlic in 2 tbsp olive oil and tamari until lightly browned and caramelized about 5-6 minutes. Then add 1/4 cup water and cook until carrots are slightly soften.

6. Then add the cooked beluga and toss together. Season with salt and pepper.

7. Then transfer to your prepared baking dish and carefully top with mashed/shredded root veggies. Smooth down with a fork and create patterns if you like.

8. Season with another crack of pepper and a little sea salt. Place on a baking sheet and bake for 12-15 minutes or until the mashers are lightly browned on top.

9. Let cool briefly before serving. The longer it sits, the more it will thicken.

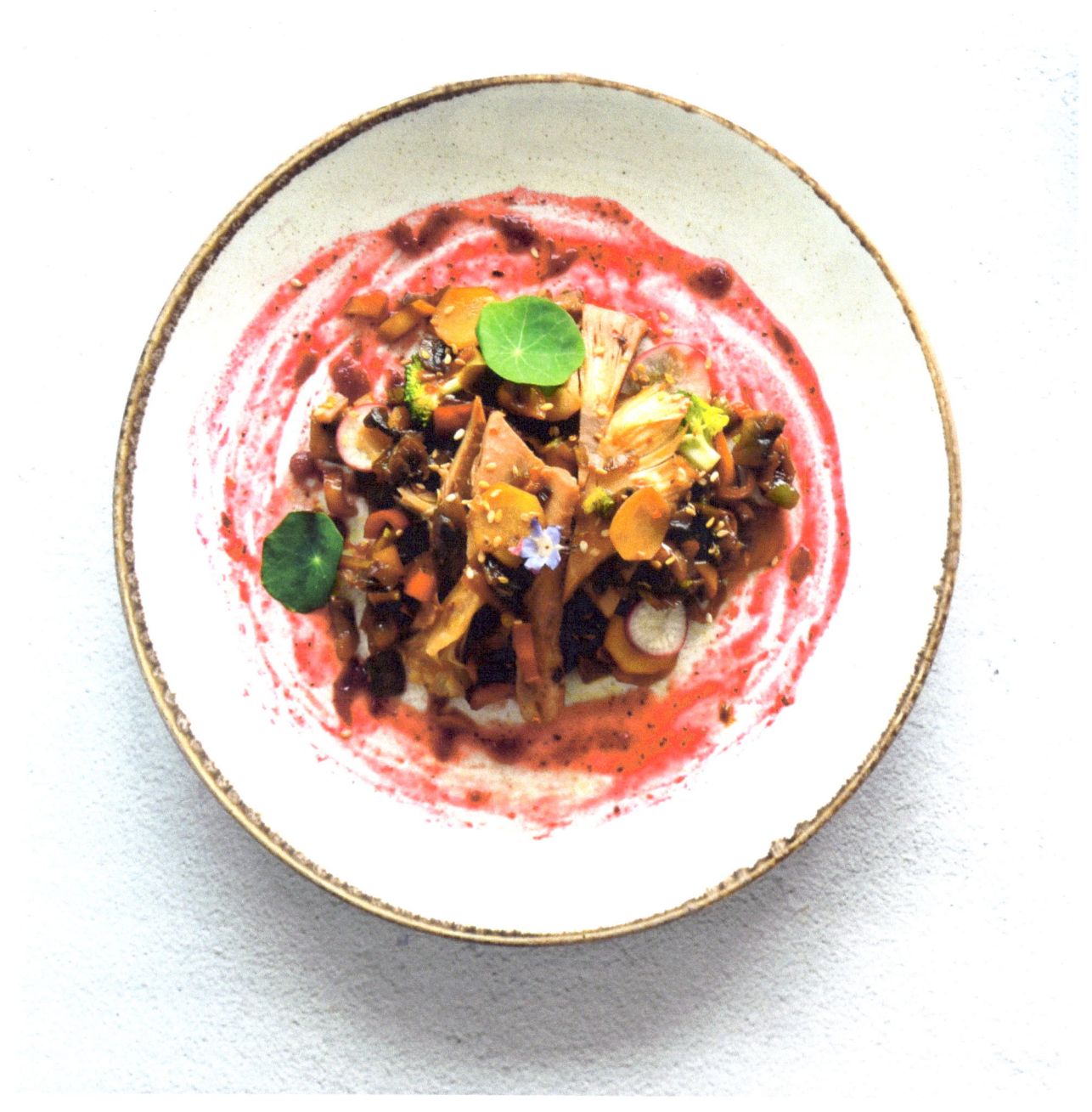

JACK IN WONDERLAND

Time - 35 minutes
Serves - 3 person

Ingredients
1/4 cup pickled red onion
4 tbsp olive oil
200 g artichoke hearts
400 g jack fruit meat
1 tsp garlic powder
1 tbsp coconut sugar
1 tsp chili powder
1 tsp thyme
1/2 tbsp apple cider vinegar
1 tsp ground mustard
1 tsp sea salt
3 tbsp tamari
1 tbsp tomato paste
2 tbsp lingon jam
1 small radish thinly sliced
1/2 cup broccoli florets steamed
Nasturtium leaves for garnish
Borage flower for garnsih
Sesame seeds to serve

1. Heat a large skillet with 3 tablespoon olive oil. Add sliced onions and sauté until caramelized.

2. Add sliced jack fruits, 1 tablespoon soy sauce and marinated artichoke hearts. Cook stirring occasionally for about 8-10 minutes on medium heat until softened and crispy.

3. In a small bow, mix garlic powder, coconut sugar, chili pepper, apple cider vinegar, thyme, mustard powder, sea salt, tamari sauce, 1 tbsp olive oil and tomato paste.

4. Pour mixture over the jack fruit artichoke mixture. Toss well until jack and artichokes are coated well. Continue to cook for 2-3 minutes. Then remove from the heat.

5. Serve with sesame seeds, lingon jam, steamed broccoli, thinly sliced radish, pickled red onion, edible flowers, nasturtium if desired.

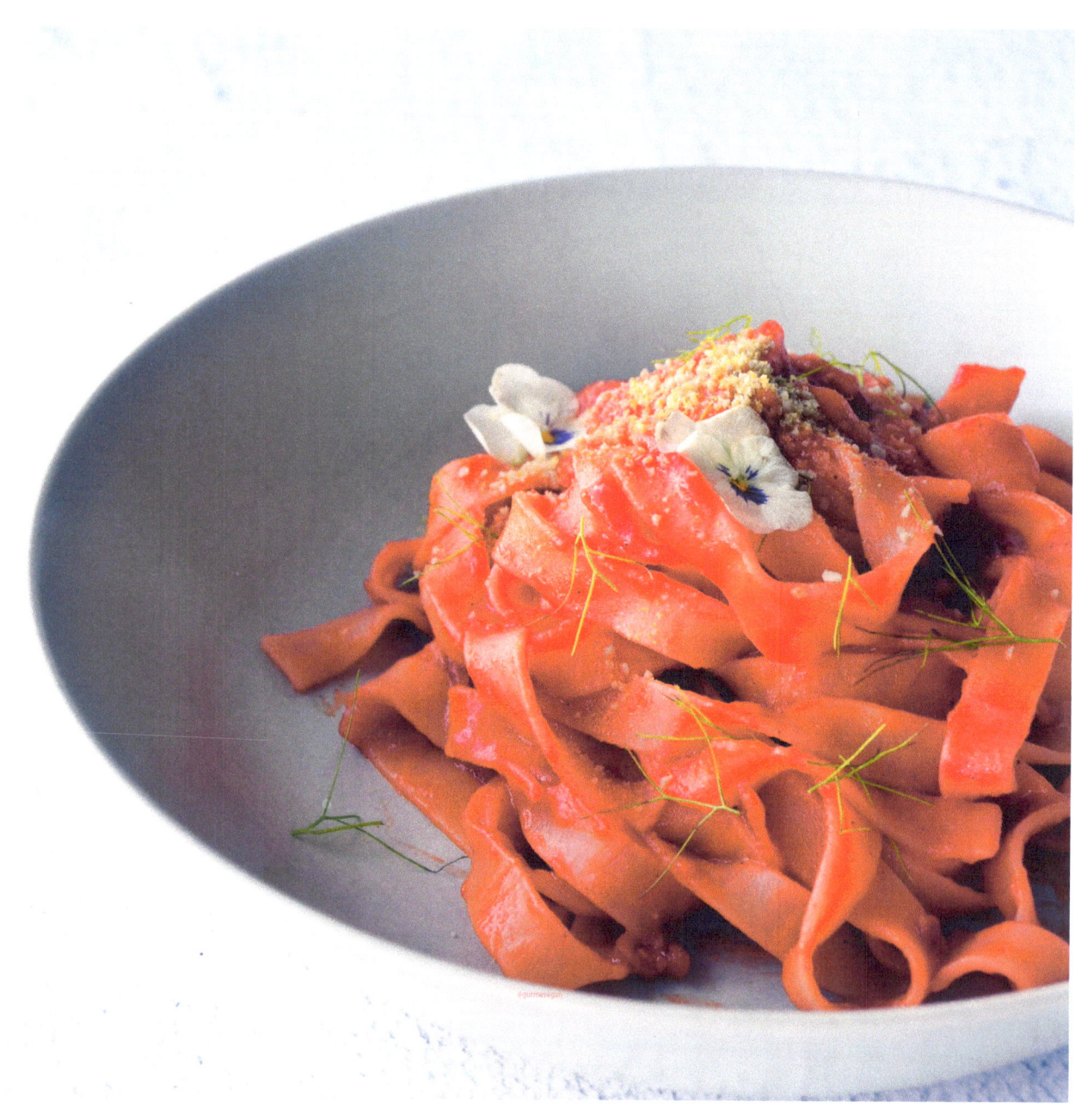

TAGLIATELLE WITH PLUM TOMATO SAUCE

Time - 30 minutes
Serves - 2

Ingredients
220 g tagliatelle
1 large damson plum (approx. 80 g)
1 large san marzano tomato (approx. 250 g)
1 spoon of tomato paste
A branch of fennel with its root
1 small carrot (optional)
2-3 cloves of garlic
2 tablespoons of olive oil
1 teaspoon of salt
1/4 teaspoon chipotle
Vegan parmesan, fennel leaves and edible flowers (optional) to serve

1. Chop the garlic and fennel into small pieces. Cook with olive oil at low heat until soft. Continue to cook until soften at a lower temperature for 2 minutes by adding vegetables and tomatoes.

2. When the tomatoes with plums soften and integrated with fennel and garlic, add the tomato paste. Then add the boiled water of the pasta around 1/4 cup. Cover the pot and cook over low to medium heat until the sauce thickens well.

3. Add the salt and chipotle and mix your sauce. If it is too dark, add more water and cook.

4. Add your cooked pasta to the sauce and toss well. Pour over 2-3 spoons of pasta water, quickly turn 3-4 times over high heat and immediately turn off the heat.

5. Divide betweeen plates. Decorate with fennel tops and sprinkle some vegan parmesan. Enjoy.

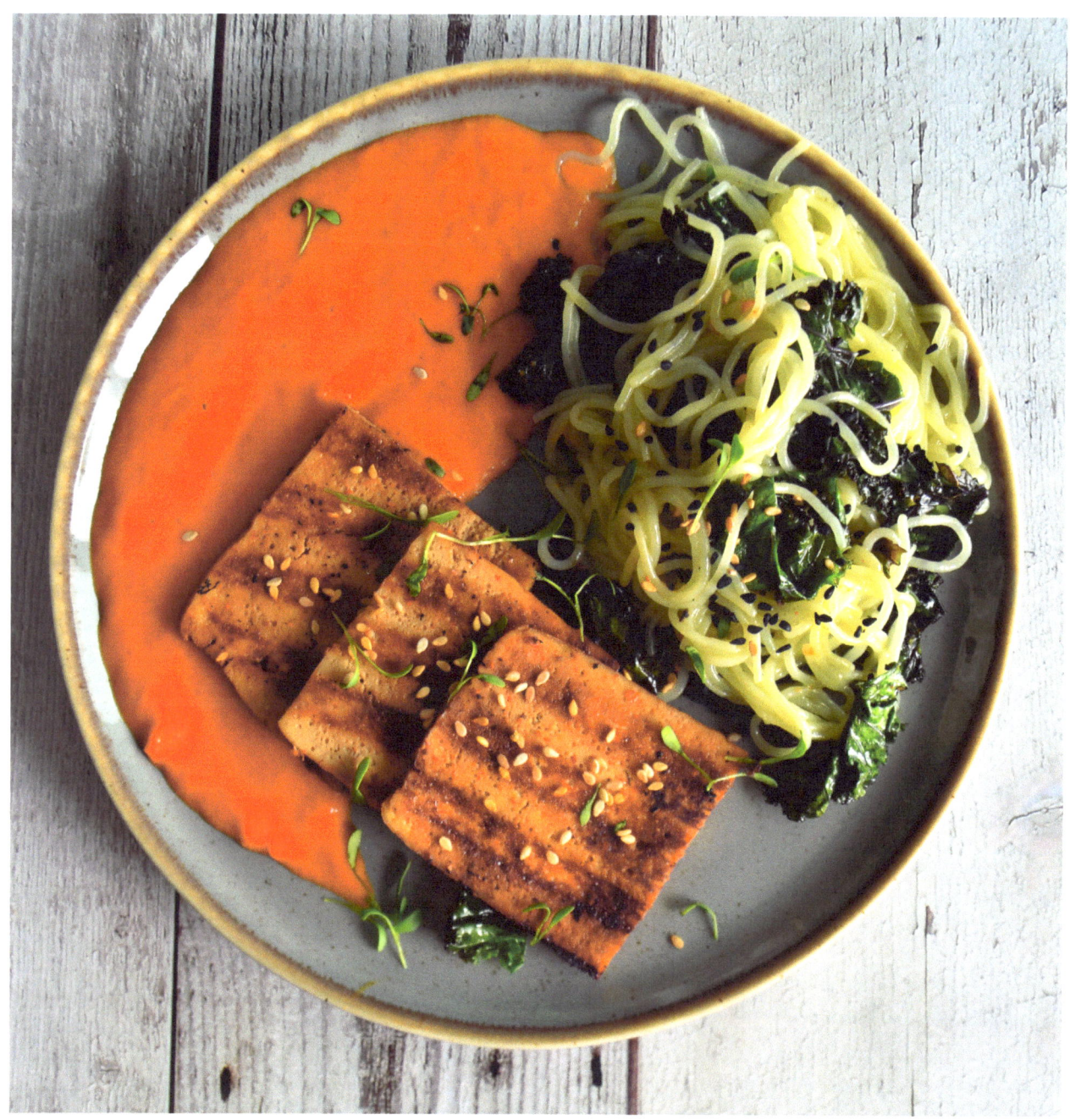

GRILLED TOFU WITH HABANERO SAUCE

Time - 45 minutes
Serves - 2-3

Ingredients
250 g firm tofu
2 tbsp lemon juice
1 tbsp maple syrup
2 tbsp tamari or soy sauce
1/4 cup porcini mushroom stock
150 ml coconut cream
1 tsp garlic powder
1 tsp chili powder
200 g konjac noodle
100 g kale leaves
1 tbsp olive oil
1 tsp sea salt
2 red bell pepper
1/2 tsp cayenne

1. To make porcini mushroom stock, add the onion, leek top, garlic, mushrooms, and salt. Give the vegetables a stir, then cover the pot and cook gently over medium heat for 15 minutes. Add the remaining ingredients and cover with 9 cups cold water. Bring the stock to a boil, then simmer, uncovered, for 1 hour.

2. In a large bowl, add mushroom stock, 1 tablespoon lemon juice, 2 tablespoons of soy sauce, 1 tablespoon maple syrup, garlic powder and chili pepper. Cut your tofu in desired shape and marinate in the sauce for about 1 hour. Roast red bell peppers at 220° C in the oven for about 22-25 minutes. Peel the skin.

3. Place peeled red bell peppers into the food processor, add coconut cream, 1 tablespoon lemon juice, soy sauce, cayenne pepper, paprika and salt. Mix on high speed until smooth. Then transfer mixture into a pot and cook on medium heat until bubbled.

4. Strain your konjac noodle, set aside. In a large skillet, heat 1 tablespoon olive oil, add kale leaves and sprinkle a bit salt. Stir-fry on high heat for 1-2 minutes. Then add konjac noodle, toss with kale leaves. Grill your marinated tofu until fried well. Pour the habanero sauce into your plate, add grilled tofu next the sauce. Add konjac noodle with kale. Sprinkle some sesame. Serve warm!

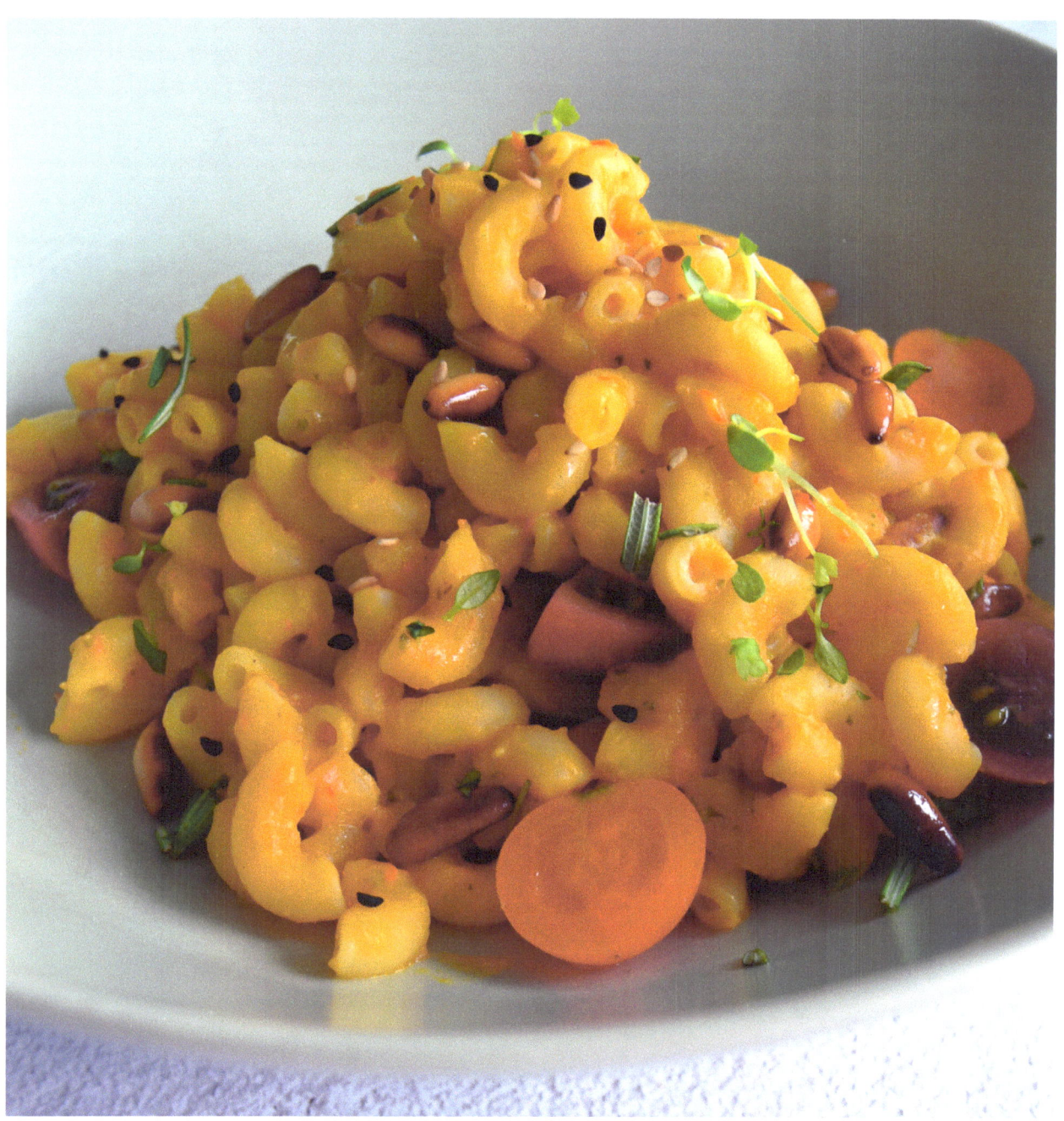

CREAMY PUMPKIN PIPETTE

Time - 40 minutes
Serves - 2

Ingredients
250 g pipette pasta
300 g butternut squash
1 large onion
1-2 tbsp olive oil
2 tsp salt
1 tsp ground mustard
25 g pine nuts
1 tbsp fresh rosemary
1 tbsp nutritional yeast
1/2 cup water + more if needed to thin
1 tsp garlic powder
1 tbsp sesame seeds
1/2 cup cherry tomatoes

1. Cook your pasta al dente, strain and set aside.

2. Cut the butternut squash into cubes, place into a mixing bowl. Cut shallots in two, add into the bowl. Sprinkle some salt, drizzle olive oil, add the mustard, nutritional yeast, garlic and rosemary. Toss everything with your hands until butternut squash coated well. Then transfer mixture onto the baking tray lined parchment paper, spread evenly.

3. Pre-heat oven to 200° C. Bake the squash in the oven for about 22-25 minutes or until roasted. Remove roasted butternut squash from the oven, place in a food processor, add 1/2 cup water. Mix on high speed until smooth. If you need, add more water to thin.

4. Pour sauce into the pot. Cook on medium heat until bubbled.

5. Then add your cooked pipette pasta and mix with the sauce.

6. Serve with cherry tomatoes, toasted pine nuts, celery micro greens and sesame seeds.

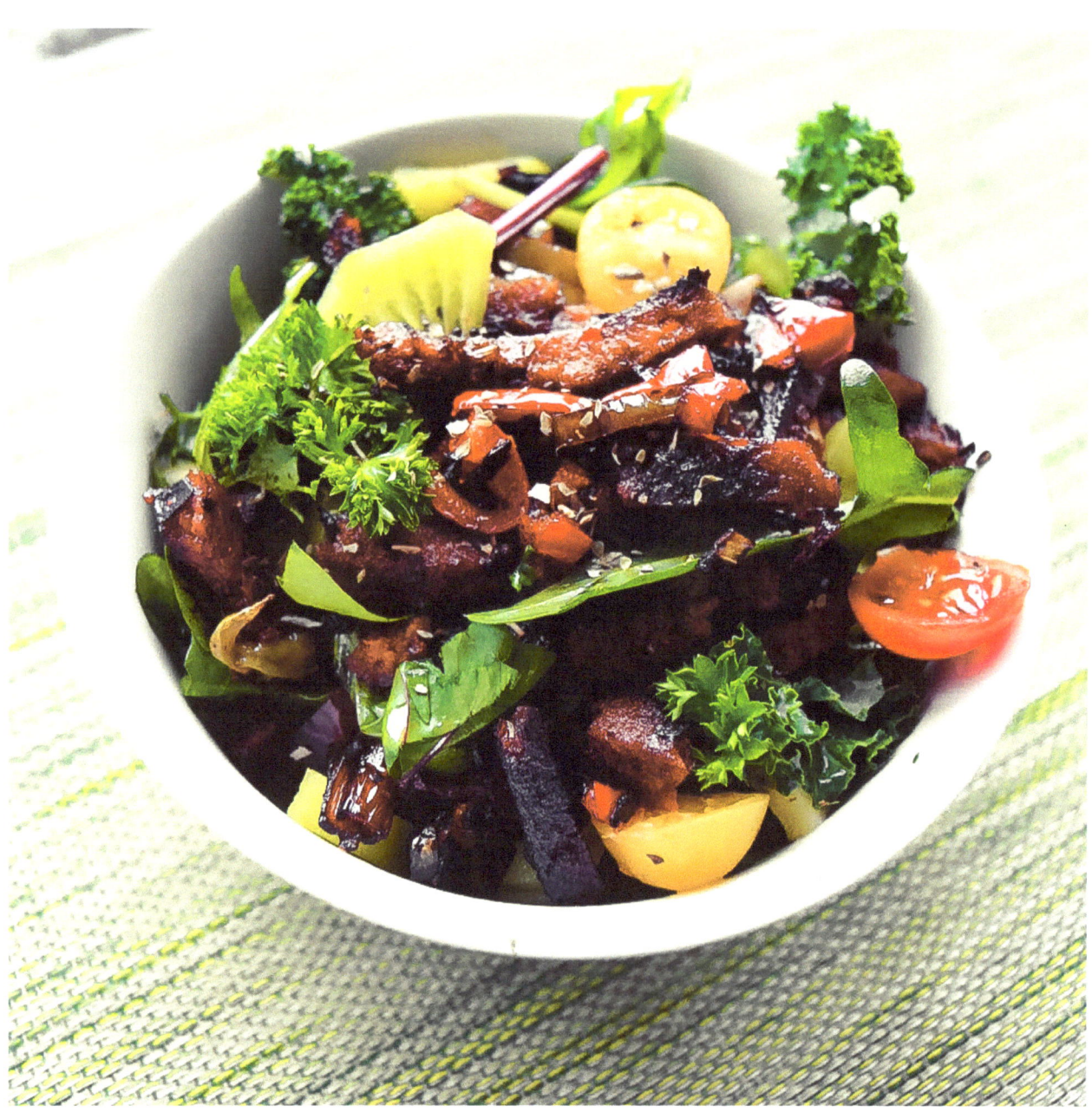

MAKING SEITAN FROM SCRATCH

Time - 2.5 hours
Serves - 2-3

Wet Ingredients

1 lt vegetable broth
2 cups water
5-6 tbsp soy sauce
4 tbsp olive oil
80 g beetroot puree
2 tbsp shiitake powder
3 tbsp vegan worcestershire

Dry Ingredients

2 cups vital gluten
1 cup chickpea flour
3 tbsp onion powder
1 tbsp garlic powder
1/4 tsp blackpepper

Glazing Ingredients

3 tbsp vegan butter
3 tbsp vegan worcestershire
1 tbsp maple syrup
2 tbsp water

Stir-Fry Ingredients

3 tbsp olive oil
3 tbsp soy sauce

1. In a large bowl, combine all dry ingredients and set aside. Place all wet ingredients in a food processor, mix on high completely smooth. Add dry ingredients into the blender, mix with the dry ingredients together.
2. Remove dough from the food processor, knead with your hands for 1-2 minutes. Give a bread shape. Pre-heat oven to 180° C. Place a baking sheet in a baking pan. Transfer dough on to the pan. Bake for 1 hour and 20 minutes. Using a large pot, bring the broth to boil.
3. When the roast is finished, place it inside the pot.
Monitor the pot frequently to make sure the broth is simmering, not boiling. Turn it every 10 minutes. Boil for 1 hour.
Refrigerate the seitan overnight to get best texture.
4. To make glazing sauce, place all sauce ingredients in a small pot, cook for 3-4 minutes on medium heat. If you need add more water or agave syrup to get sticky sauce.
Next morning, spread sauce over the seitan. Let it cool at least 30 min. Cut into small long pieces or cubes. Heat stir fry ingredients; olive oil and soy sauce in large pan, add seitan pieces, stir-fry on high heat until crispy. Serve with your favorite greens and nuts.

Liquid Tips:
to turn seitan into dark color, use more soy sauce and vegetable broth.
to make a soft texture, use only water.
to make spicy and intense seitan, use more soy sauce and peppers.

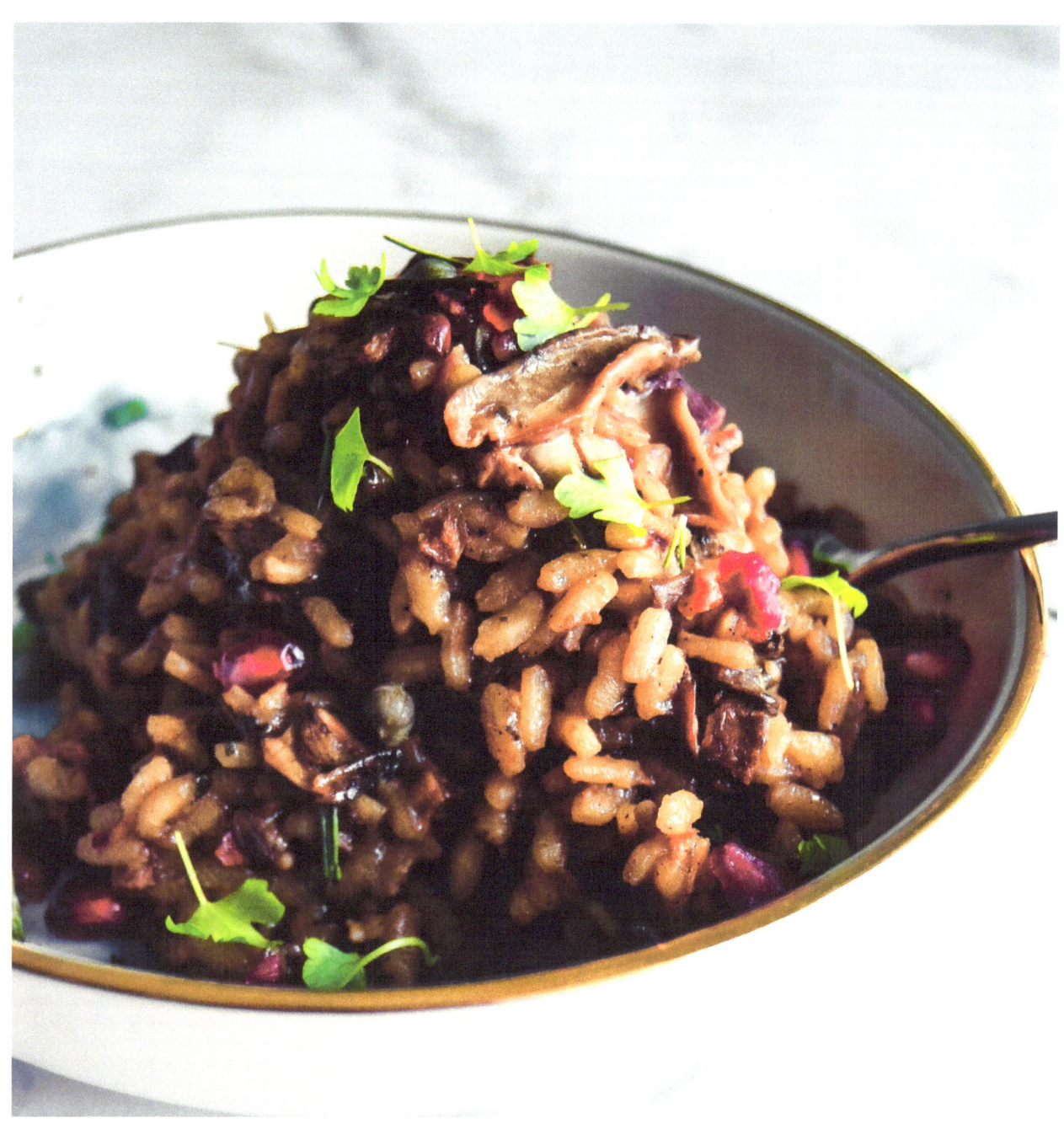

RISOTTO WITH MUSHROOMS AND POMEGRANATES

Time - 30 minutes
Serves - 2

Ingredients
1 cup risotto rice
2 shallot
1 cup porcini mushrooms
1/2 cup pomegranates
2 tbsp olive oil
1/2 cup vegetable stock
2 tbsp tamari or soy sauce
1/2 cup oat cream
1 bay leaf
1/4 cup vegan white wine
1/2 tsp fresh thyme
Salt and pepper to taste
1 tbsp vegan butter
Parsley microgreens to serve
Vegan parmesan to serve

1. Soak dried porcini in 3 cups water until rehydrated, about an hour. Strain the mushrooms, reserving the broth for the risotto. (Discard the last 1/2 inch of the liquid; it will contain dirt from the porcini.) Roughly chop the mushrooms, then set aside. When you're ready, heat the vegetable stock and mushroom broth to a simmer.
2. In a large saucepan, heat 2 tablespoons of the oil and tamari until shimmering. Add the shallot and garlic and cook over moderate heat, stirring, until softened, 2 minutes. Add the risotto rice and dried porcini and stir to coat.
3. Add the wine and bay leaf and cook until the wine has evaporated. Add about one-fourth of the warm stock and cook over moderate heat, stirring constantly, until nearly absorbed. Continue adding the stock in batches, stirring constantly until the rice is al dente and suspended in a creamy sauce, about 20 minutes. Discard the bay leaf. Stir in the vegan butter, oat cream and vegan cheese; season with salt and pepper and keep warm.
4. In a skillet, heat the remaining 2 tablespoons of oil. Add the fresh porcini and thyme and cook over high heat, stirring, until softened and golden, 8 minutes. Discard the thyme. Season the porcini with salt and pepper, spoon over the risotto and serve with pomegranates and celery microgreens.

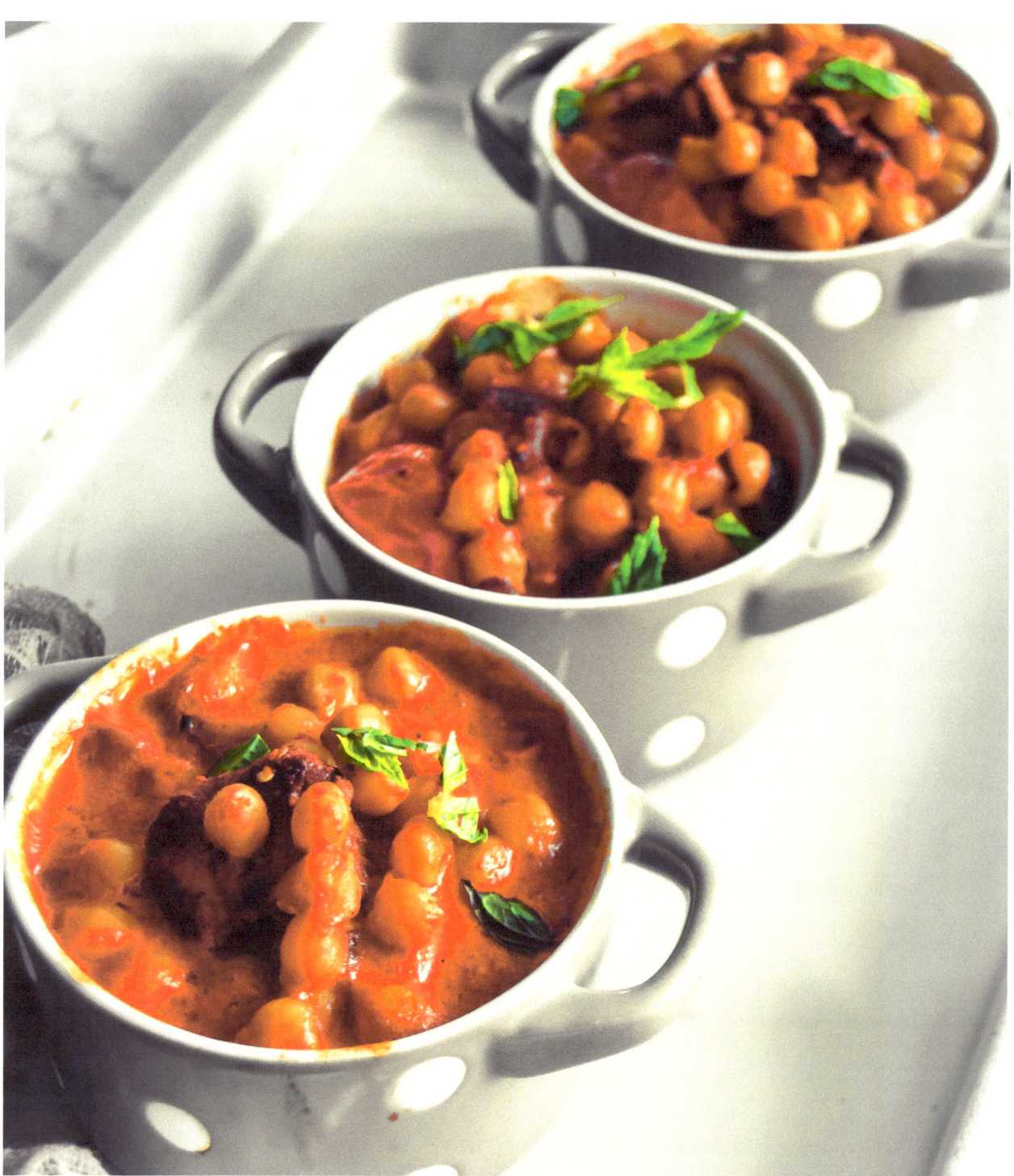

CREAMY CHICKPEA CURRY WITH CHANTERELLES

Time - 1 hour
Serves - 2-3

Ingredients

1 cup chanterelle mushrooms
1 cup chickpeas soaked overnight
1 cup cherry tomatoes
2 red bell peppers chopped
1 red onion chopped
1 tbsp olive oil
2 garlic cloves minced
2 tbsp tamari or soy sauce
220 ml coconut milk
1/2 tsp salt
3 tbsp nutritional yeast
1/2 tsp curry powder
2 tbsp lemon juice
1/2 tsp paprika
1/4 tsp dried rosemary
Fresh mint for garnish

1. Pre-heat oven to 200° C.

2. Place the chickpeas in a pot, cover with water. Bring to boil until soften.

3. Heat a large skillet pan, saute onion, red bell peppers and garlic in olive oil until golden brown.

4. Then add the coconut milk, tomatoes, red peppers, curry, nutritional yeast, salt and smoked paprika, rosemary, lemon juice, tamari and chanterelles. Cook on high heat until thicken.

5. Lastly add cooked chickpeas in the pot, stir well in the mushrooms and continue to cook for about 2-3 mintes.

6. Transfer mixture in small bowls. Bake in the oven until thicken and tops are golden brown.

7. Serve with vegan parmesan and mint if desired.
.

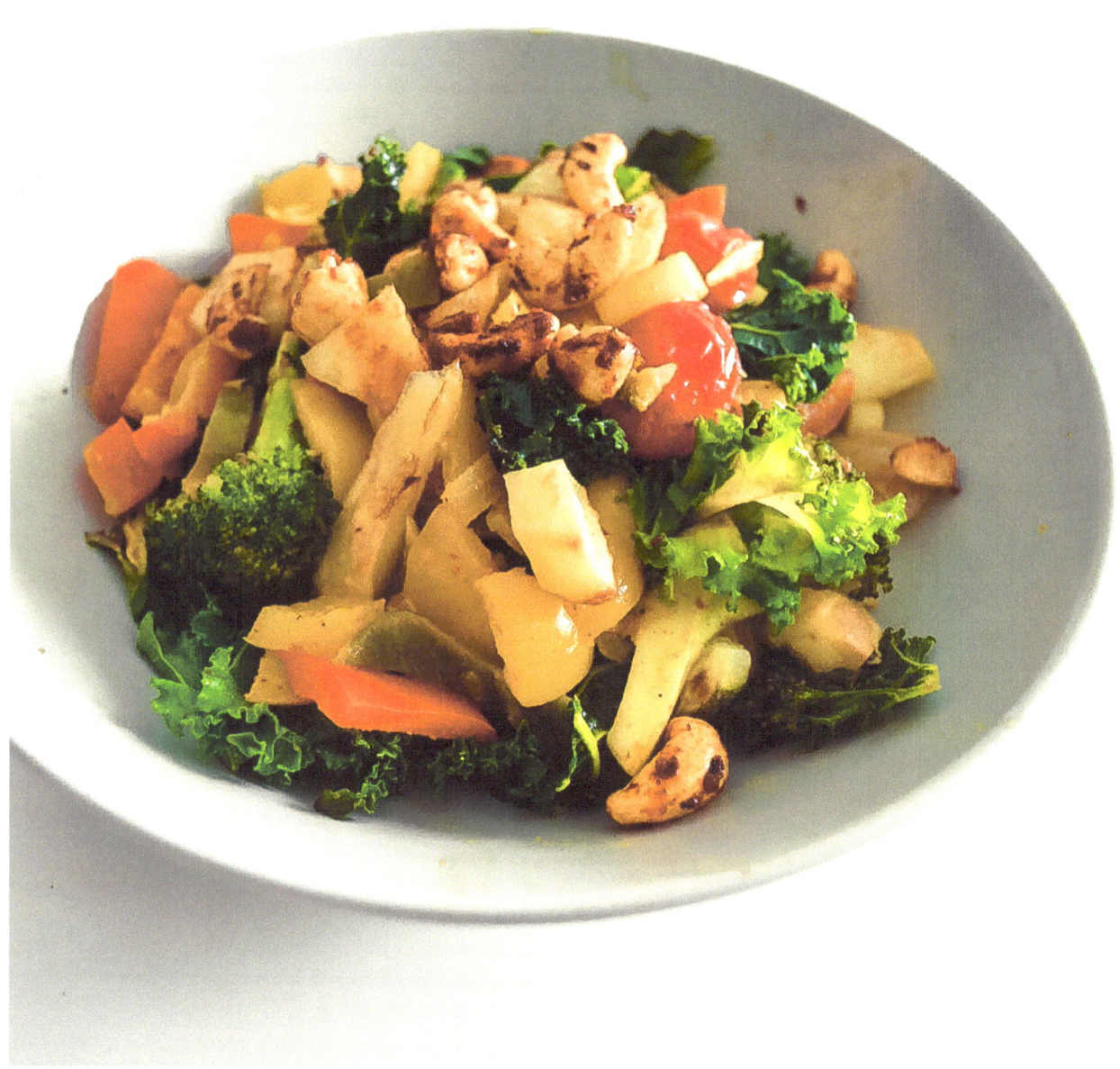

POTATO CURRY WITH KALE AND NUTS

Time - 1 hour
Serves - 2

Ingredients
2 medium potatoes
1 large zucchini
100 g kale
4 tbsp olive oil
2-3 bell peppers
1 onion chopped
1 tsp ginger powder
1 tsp coriander
1/4 cup tangerine or orange juice
2 tsp curry powder
1 cup cherry tomatoes
1 small broccoli head
60 g cashews

1. Pre-heat oven to 200° C. Peel and cut potatoes and zucchini into chunks. Place onto the baking tray with parchment paper. Pour 1 tbsp olive oil over them. Roast for 30-40 minutes until golden.

2. To make vegetable mix, chop broccoli, onions and yellow, red, green capsicums and add them into a pan, caramelize with 2 tbsp olive oil for 5-6 minutes.

3. To make curry sauce, in a small bowl mix coriander, curry, salt, tangerine juice and ginger.

4. Place kale pieces in a large pan, drizzle 1 tbsp oil, and pour 1 tbsp curry mix sauce over them. Toss on high heat for 3-4 minutes. Set aside. Pour remaining curry sauce over the vegetable mix, stir and mix well.

5. In a small pan, mix cashews with 1 tsp chili pepper and 1 tbsp oil until toasted well.

6. Remove baking tray from the oven, let cool for 10-15 minutes.

7. Place roasted zucchini and potatoes in a plate. Add vegetable mix and kale leaves. Top with cashews. Serve with cooked quinoa or black wild rice for a filling meal if desired.

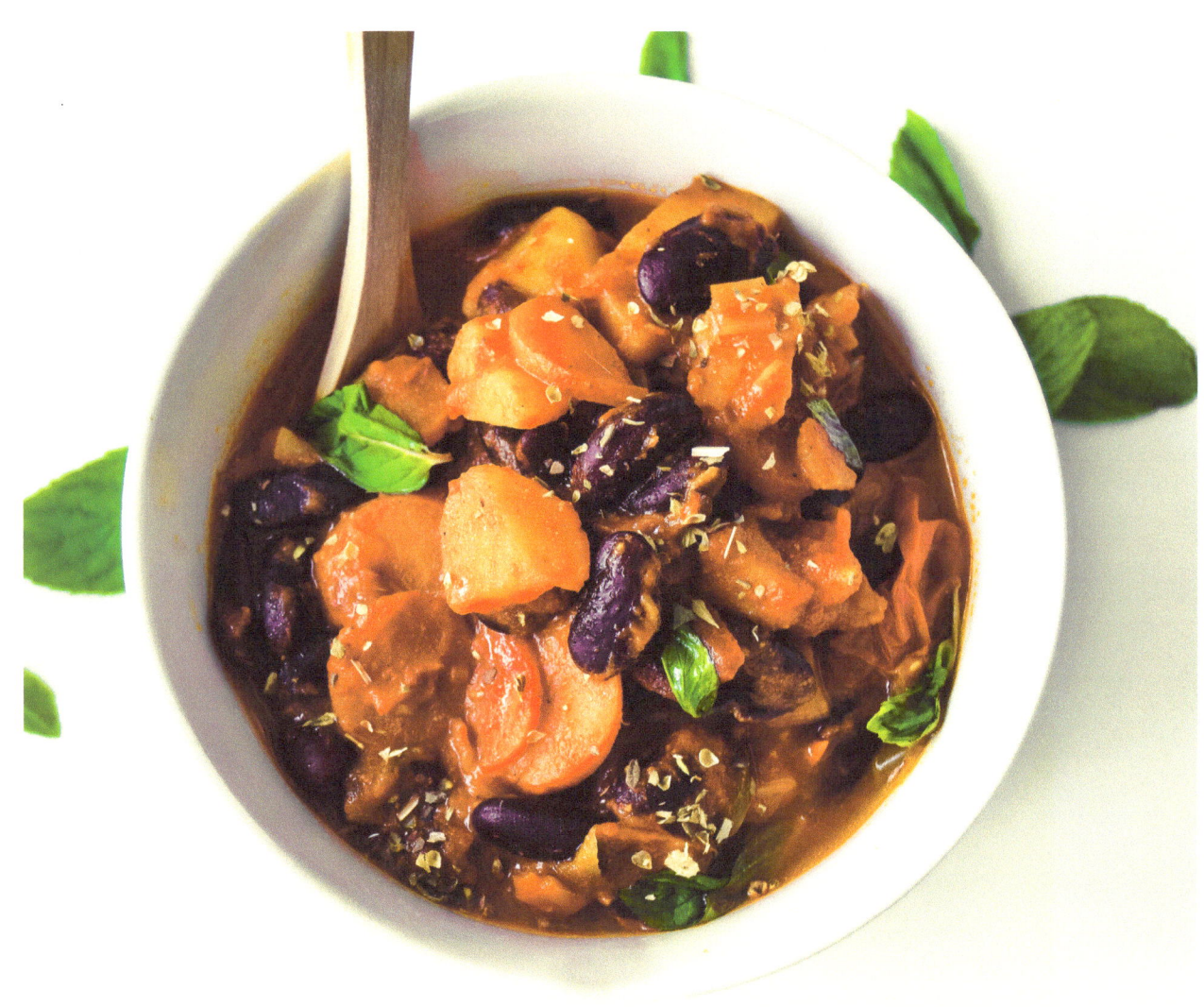

CHIPOTLE BLACK BEANS

Time - 1 hour
Serves - 2-3

Ingredients
200 g black beans
1 tbsp olive oil
1 leek
1 carrot
2 small potatoes
1 jalapeno
1/4 cup vegetable stock
1 tbsp nutritional yeast
1 tsp salt
1 tsp garlic
1 tsp ground mustard
1 tbsp tomato paste
175 g cherry tomatoes
1 tsp chipotle powder

1. Wash your beans, place in a deep pot, cover with water. Bring to boil until lightly soft. Strain and set aside.

2. In a large pan, heat olive oil, add chopped leeks, carrots, potatoes, jalapeno. Saute until caramelized.

3. Then add the cherry tomatoes, garlic, mustard, tomato paste chili powder, salt and nutritional yeast. Stir and add 200ml. water.

4. Cook on medium heat for 5 minutes. Then add vegetable cube, chipotle spice, beans and cook until lightly softened. Cook on medium heat for 10 minutes.

5. Pre-heat oven to 200° C.

6. Transfer everything into a dutch oven. Roast for 15-20 minutes or until golden browned. Let it cool for 15 minutes before serving. Top with fresh mint leaves or parsley if desired. Serve with rice for a filling meal.

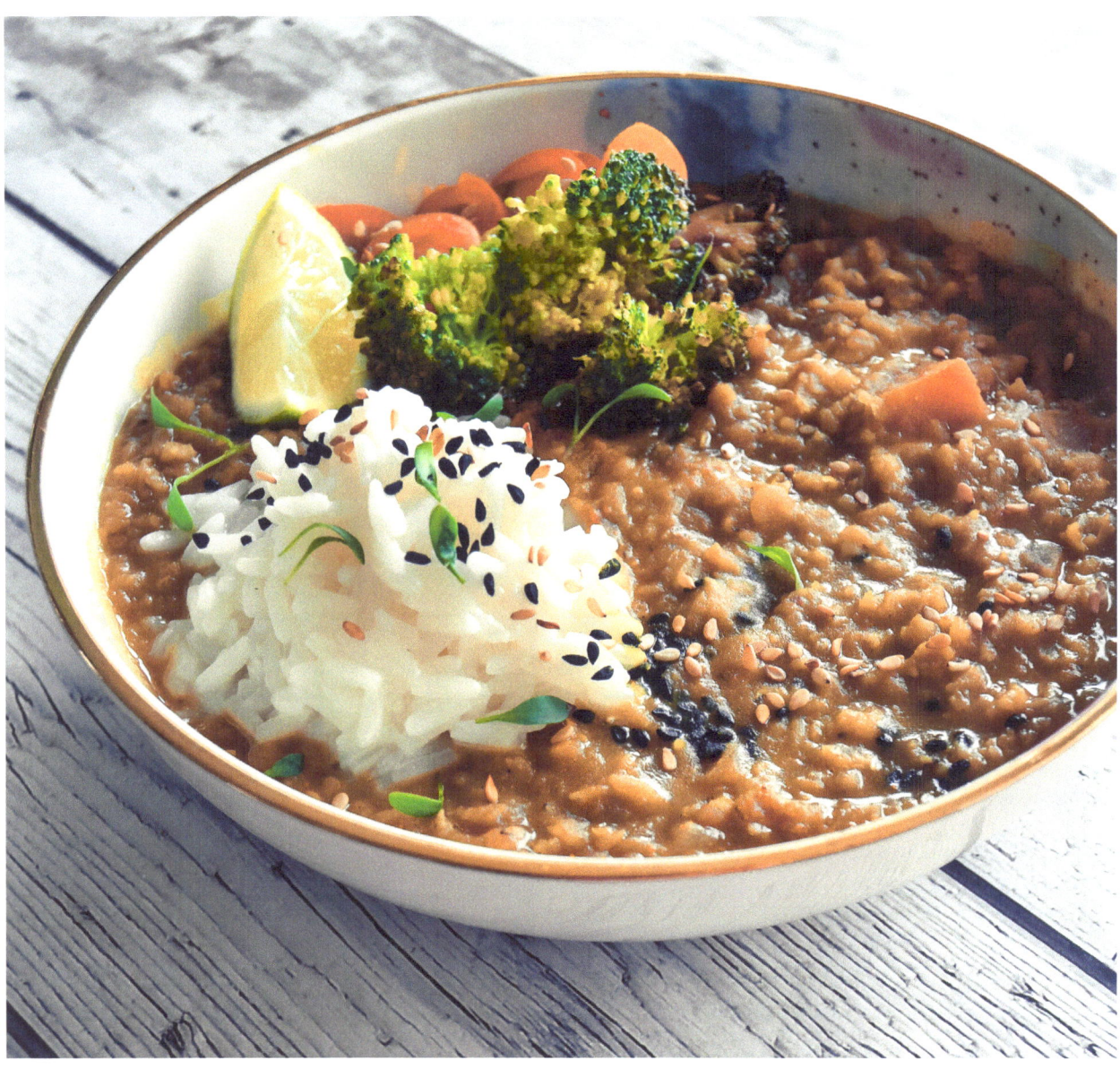

RED LENTIL DAHL WITH BUTTERNUT SQUASH CREAM

Time - 45 minutes
Serves - 2

Ingredients
1 cup red lentil
100 g butternut squash cubed
2 garlic cloves minced
1 red onion chopped
1 tsp ground ginger
1/2 cup coconut milk
1 tsp curry powder
1 cup vegetable stock
1 tbsp tamari or soy sauce
1/2 tsp cayenne
1 tsp ground coriander
1/2 head broccoli florets
1 cup cherry tomatoes

1. Heat oil in a saucepan over a medium heat. Cook onions for 5-6 minutes until tender. Add garlic and curry powder. Cook for 2 minutes or until fragrant.

2. Add the lentils, butternut cubes, ginger, coriander, coconut milk, cayenne, salt and stock. Bring to the boil. Reduce heat to low. Simmer, partially covered, for 30 minutes or until lentils have softened and thick. Remove from heat.

3. In a large skillet pan, heat olive oil and tamari, add broccoli florets and occasionally stirring, cook broccoli on high heat until gets color.

4. Place the red lentil dahl to your bowl, add the broccoli and cherry tomatoes. Serve warm with rice and lemon if desired.

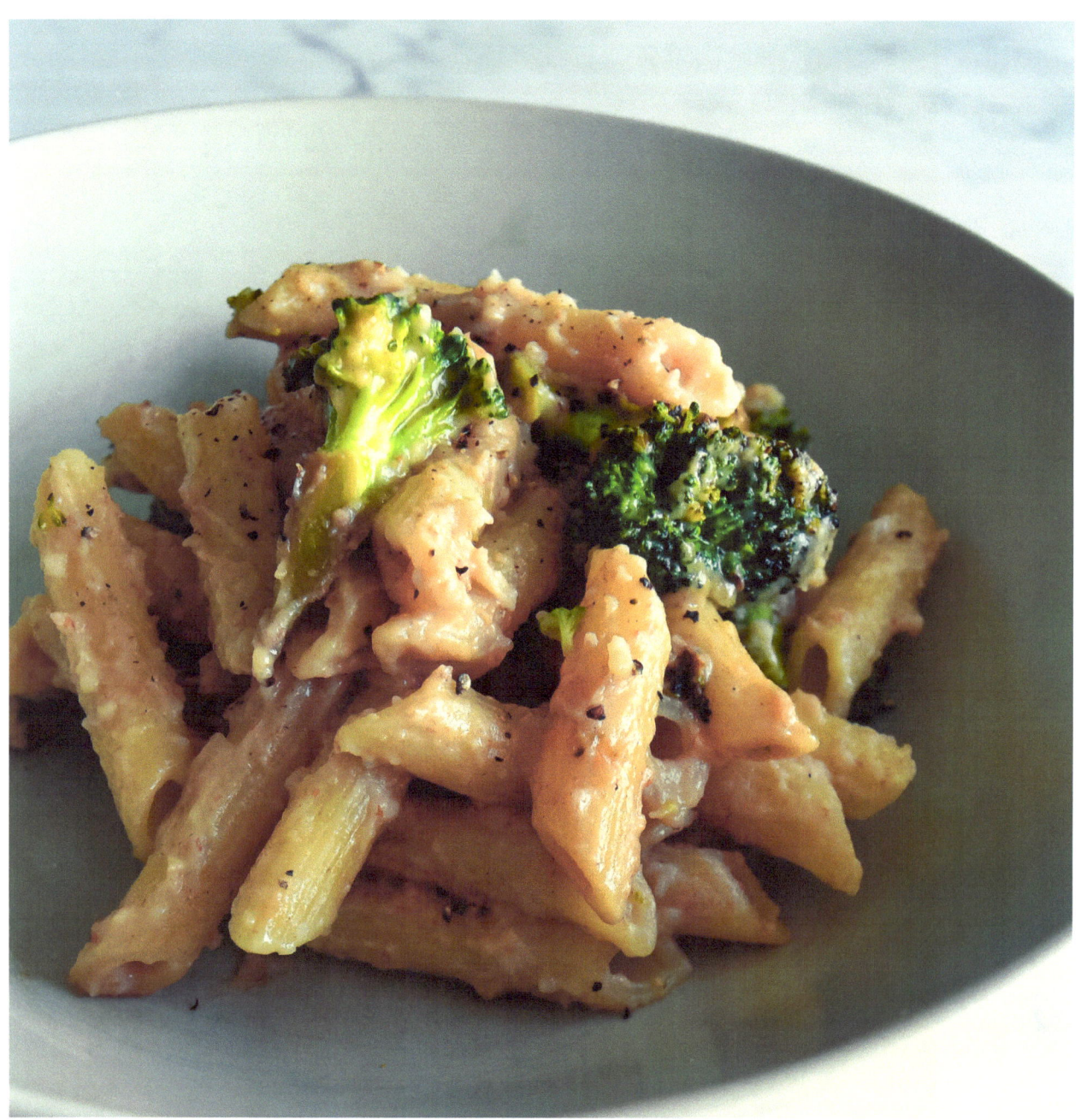

PENNE WITH ALFREDO SAUCE AND BROCCOLI

Time - 35 minutes
Serves - 2

Ingredients
3 tbsp vegan butter
3 tbsp flour
2 cups oat milk
3 tbsp nutritional yeast
250 g penne
1/2 tsp garlic powder
1/4 tsp onion powder
1 tsp salt
2 tbsp tamari
2 tbsp olive oil
2 cups broccoli florets
Salt and pepper to taste

1. Soak 1 cup oats in purified water for at least 30 minutes, After soaking, drain and rinse the oats well. Put soaked, rinsed, drained oats into blender, add 3 cups of purified water. Blend and strain in a nut milk bag to remove pulp.

2. In a medium pan, heat oil on medium heat. Add flour slowly. Cook for 1-2 minutes, continue to whisk until smooth. Then add the oat milk, salt, garlic, onion powder and nutritional yeast. Turn heat to medium-low and cook until thicken.

3. Cook your pasta according to package and set aside.

4. Heat a larg skillet pan, add olive oil and tamari. Stir-fry broccoli florets on high heat for 2-3 minutes.

5. Transfer broccoli florets into the oat sauce.

6. Add pasta into the pot. Toss well together. Serve warm.

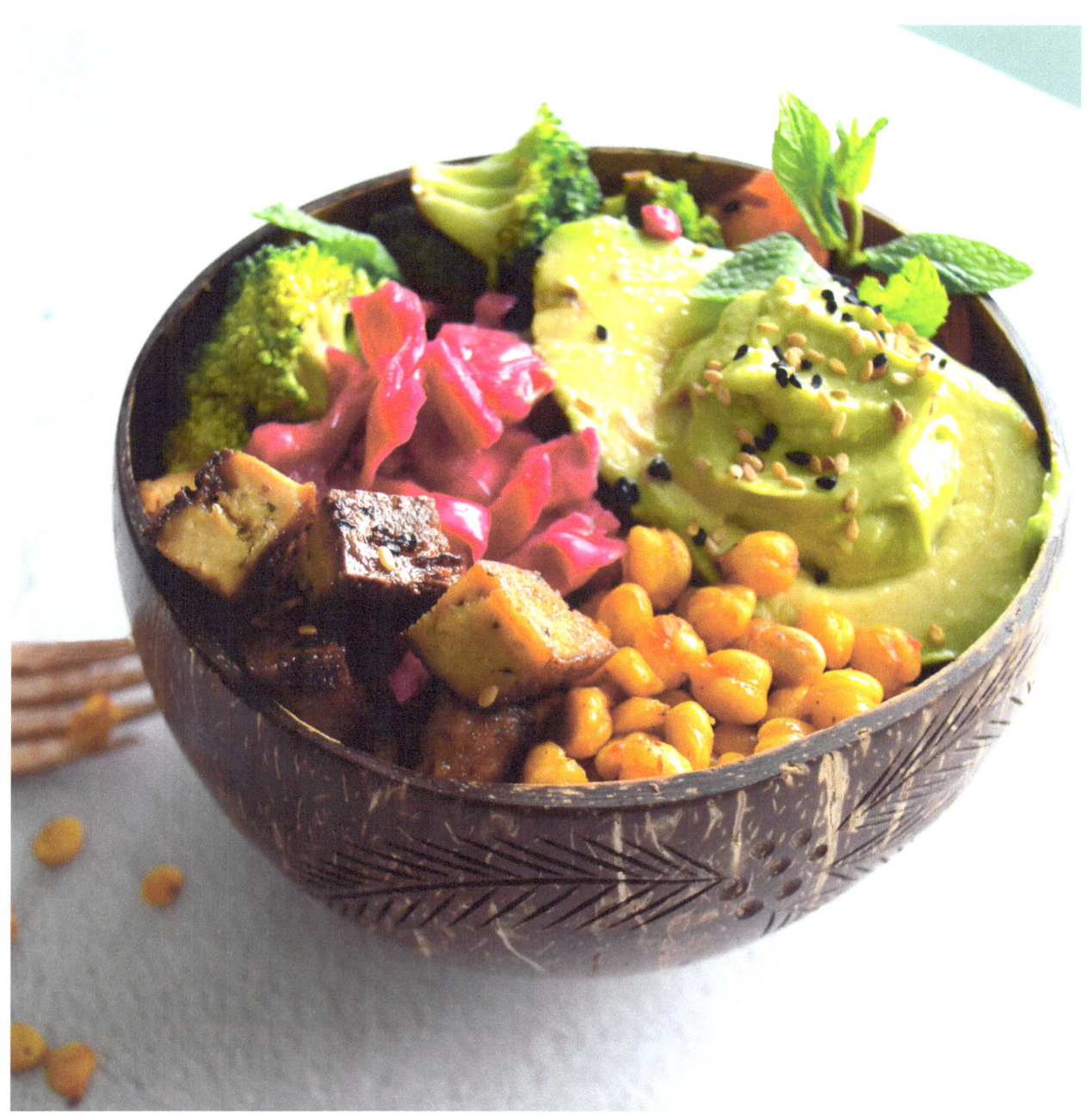

BUDDHA BOWL

Time - 1 hour
Serves - 2

Ingredients
1 ripe avoado
1-2 tbsp lemon juice
1 garlic clove minced
1 cup toasted chickpeas
1/4 tsp cayenne
1/4 tsp thyme
1/4 tsp rosemary
200 g firm tofu
3 tbsp tamari
2 tbsp olive oil
1/4 cup pickled red cabbage
1/4 cup pickled red onion
1 cup steamed broccoli
Fresh mint or parsley
1 cup cherry tomatoes
Salt and pepper to taste

1. Peel and core your avocado, place the half in a blender, add 1-2 tbsp lemon juice, a pinch salt and 1 garlic clove minced. Mix together until creamy. Then place the cream in the middle of the other half of the avocado. (if you want to serve this way, otherwise it is just ok to slice and put in the bowl.)

2. Place precooked chickpeas in a bowl, drizzle some olive oil, 1/4 tsp cayenne, thyme, rosemary, pepper and salt. Toss together. Place on a baking tray lined parchment paper. Bake in the oven at 200° C until crispy. Then transfer to your buddha bowl.

3. To steam your broccoli, pour about an inch of water into a skillet or wok and bring it to a boil over medium-high heat. Put the broccoli florets in a steamer basket and season with salt. Set the steamer basket over boiling water and cook until the broccoli is crisp-tender, 8 to 10 minutes depending on the size of the florets. Add the your buddha bowl.

4. Cut your tofu into cubes, drizzle 2 tbsp olive oil and 3 tbsp tamari. Place in the oven, bake at 200° C until crispy or fry in the pan. Then add to your buddha bowl.

5. Add the pickled cabbage, onion, halved tomatoes and fresh herbs. Serve.

SWEETS

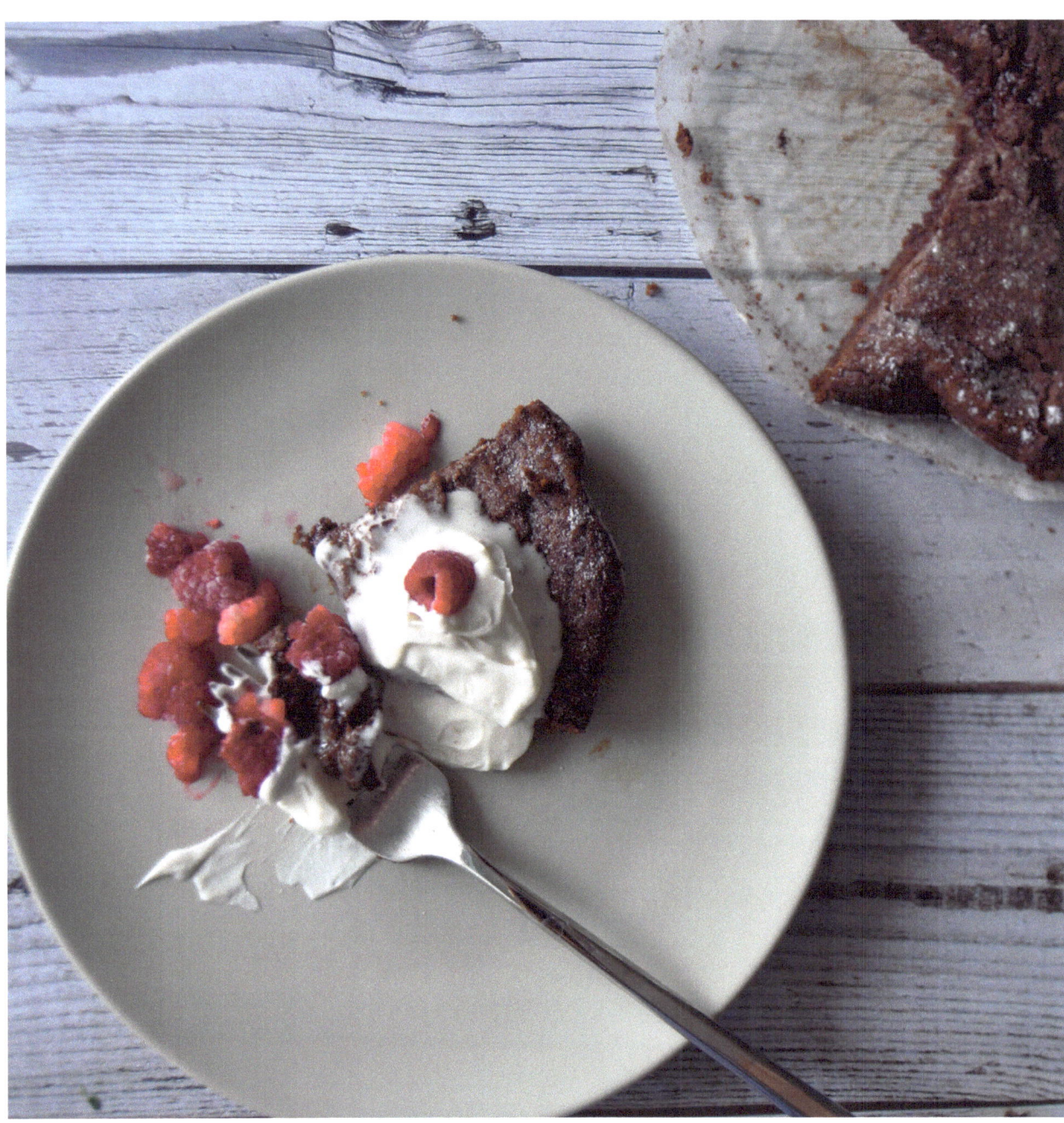

KLADDKAKA
SWEDISH STYLE STICKY BROWNIE

Time - 30 minutes
Serves - 4-5

Ingredients

2 tsp lupin powder or ground flaxseed + 60 ml water
100 g vegan butter or coconut oil melted
140 g coconut sugar
40 g maple syrup
150 g all purpose flour
4 tbsp cacao powder
1-2 tbsp plant milk + more as needed
1 tsp vanilla powder
A pinch salt

One of the most popular baked goods in Sweden is the kladdkaka. Kladdkaka is just gooey, chocolate yumminess, kind of like brownies.
Swedish brownies are called "kladdkaka" in Swedish which means sticky cake. I definitely recommend it with oat or coconut cream or ice cream on the top. It isn't as dense as a regular cake, it is soft and fudgy.

1. To make, in a large bowl, whisk egg replacer (lupin powder or grounf flax) , water, coconut sugar and vegan butter together until fluffy.
Meanwhile pre-heat oven to 190° C.
2. Add the flour, vanilla and salt into the bowl, mix on high speed until completely smooth mixture.
3. Use a 16 cm spring-roll pan , dust it with cacao powder.
4. Pour mixture into the pan.
5. Bake for 20 minutes. Keep on eye on the cake in order to prevent baking too much.
 6. Let it cool at least 1 hour and then cut into slices, sprinkle icing sugar, serve with whipped cream, icecream and your favorite forest berries.

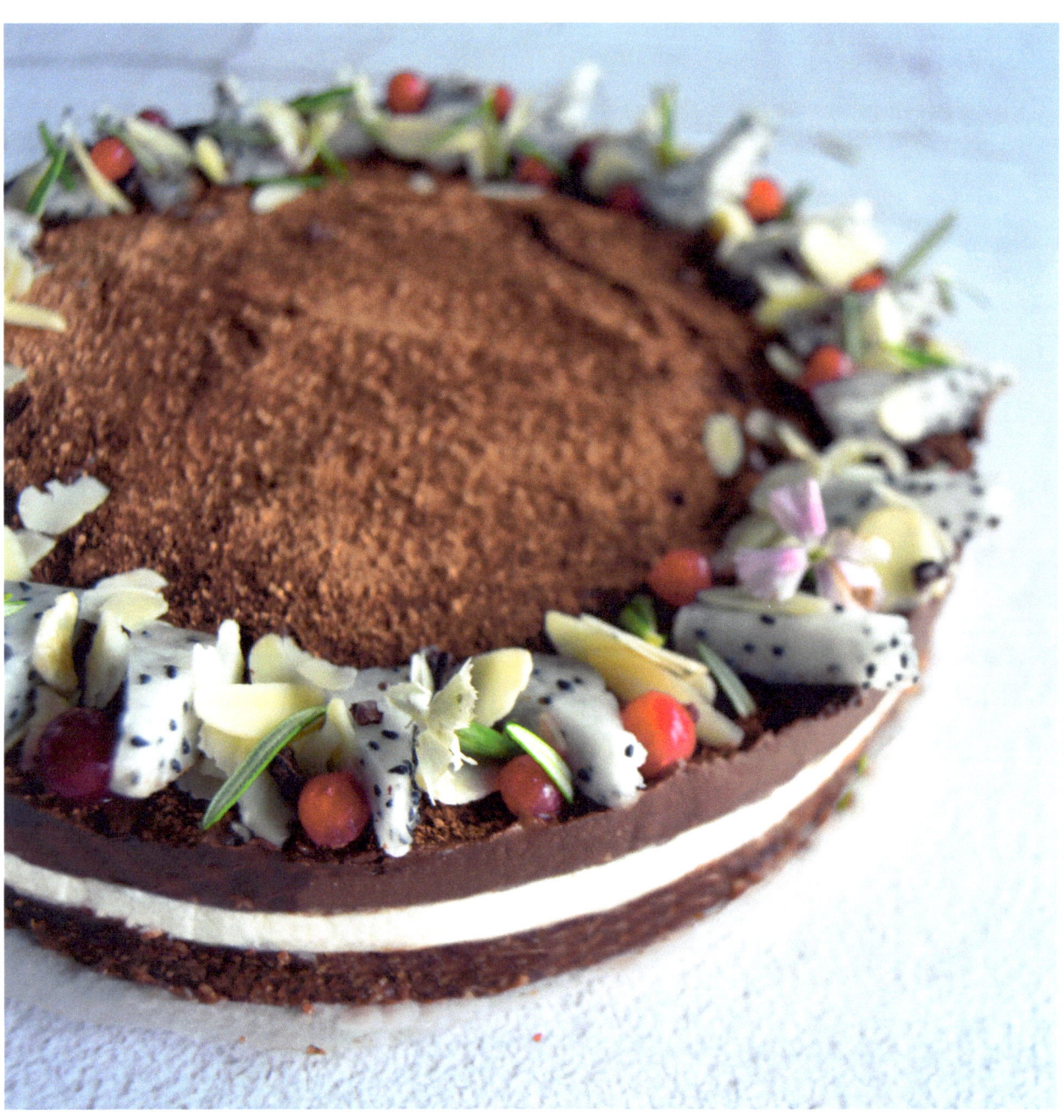

THREE LAYER FESTIVE RAW CAKE

Time - 50 minutes + 4 hrs setting
Serves - 6-8

Crust
60 g oat flour
60 g hazelnut meal
50 g raw cacao powder
100 g fresh medjool dates pitted
30 g maple syrup
1/4 tsp salt
1-2 tbsp almond milk + more as needed until everything holds together

Cream Layer
120 g raw cashews soaked
1/4 cup coconut cream (only fatty part)
2 tbsp lemon juice
3 tbsp maple syrup
3 tbsp coconut oil melted

Chocolate Layer
1 ripe avocado peeled and cored
175 g vegan dark chocolate melted
2 tbsp raw cacao powder
1 tbsp maple syrup
1-2 tbsp coconut milk to thin
A pinch salt

For garnish
Lingonberries pitaya, rosemary, edible flowers, sliced almonds, raw cacao to dust.

1. To make crust, place the oat flour, hazelnut meal, raw cacao and salt into your food processor, process until everything combined well. Then add the fresh medjool dates (if not fresh, then soak in the water and strain before using), maple syrup and almond milk. Process again, add more almond milk if needed. The dough should be sticky and holds together. Once done, transfer to a spring pan about 16-18 cm lined parchment paper. Press down and spread the dough evenly. Set aside.

2. Place your cashews in a bowl, cover with water, soak for 4-5 hours. Then strain and dry. Transfer to the blender. Add the lemon juice, coconut cream and maple. Blend until you get silky smooth cream. Lastly add the melted coconut oil. Blend again.
Pour mixture over the crust. Let it sit in the fridge while you are making the chocolate layer.

3. Peel your avocado, remove the seed. Transfer the meat in the food processor. Add the melted vegan dark chocolate (melt using bain marie method beforehand.) , raw cacao powder, maple syrup, coconut milk and a pinch of salt. Process until everything combined well and you get a silky smooth mixture.

4. Remove the cake from the freezer, pour the chocolate cream over the white cream layer. Place in the freezer again for about 4 hours.

5. Once time is up, remove from the freezer and cake mould. Dust some raw cacao, decorate with fruits, nuts and herbs.

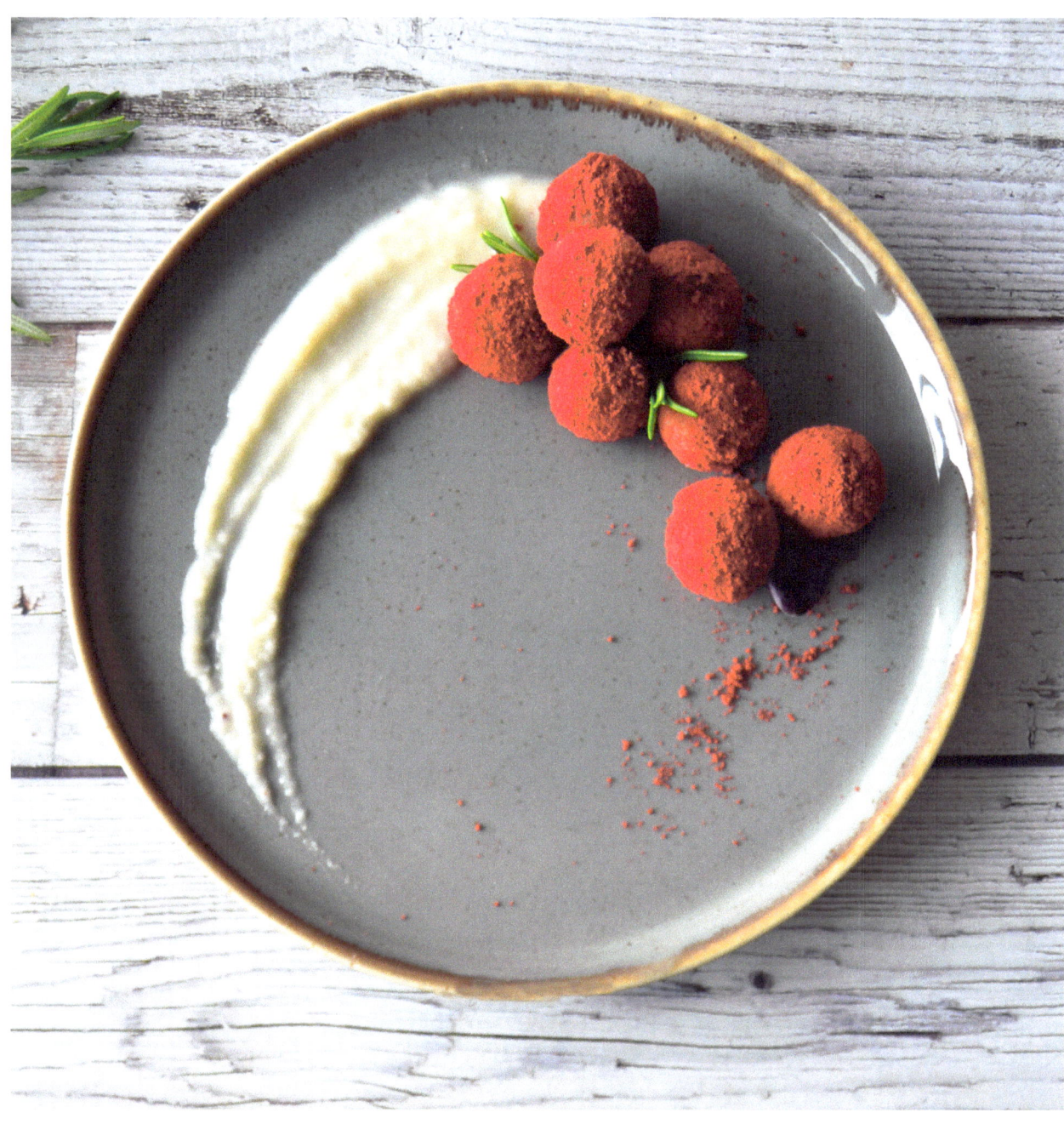

LINGON DONUT BALLS WITH MACADAMIA CREAM

Time - 40 minutes
Serves - 4 plates

Ingredients
2 cup almond flour
1 cup organic coconut flour
3 tbsp coconut nectar or maple
2 tsp vanilla extract
200 g medjool dates
1 lemon juice
4 tbsp coconut oil

Macadamia Cream
100 g raw macadamia nuts pre-soaked
3 tbsp coconut cream
2 tbsp raw cacao butter melted
2 tbsp lemon juice
3 tbsp maple syrup
1/2 tsp vanilla extract

lingonberry powder for coating
fresh rosemary for garnish

1. Soak dates in warm water for about 15-20 minutes.

2. Then add to the food processor, mix on high for about 2-3 minutes.

3. Add almond flour, coconut flour, coconut nectar or maple, vanilla extract, cardamom, lemon juice and coconut oil into your blender.

4. Mix on high speed until you get dough texture.

5. Remove dough from the blender. Make small balls with your hands.

6. Coat with lingonberry powder.

7. Add soaked, rinsed macadamia nuts into the food processor, add all remaining macadamia cream ingredients, mix on high speed until silky smooth.

8. Spread the macadamia cream on the plate. Place balls over cream. Decorate with fresh rosemary leaves. Serve.

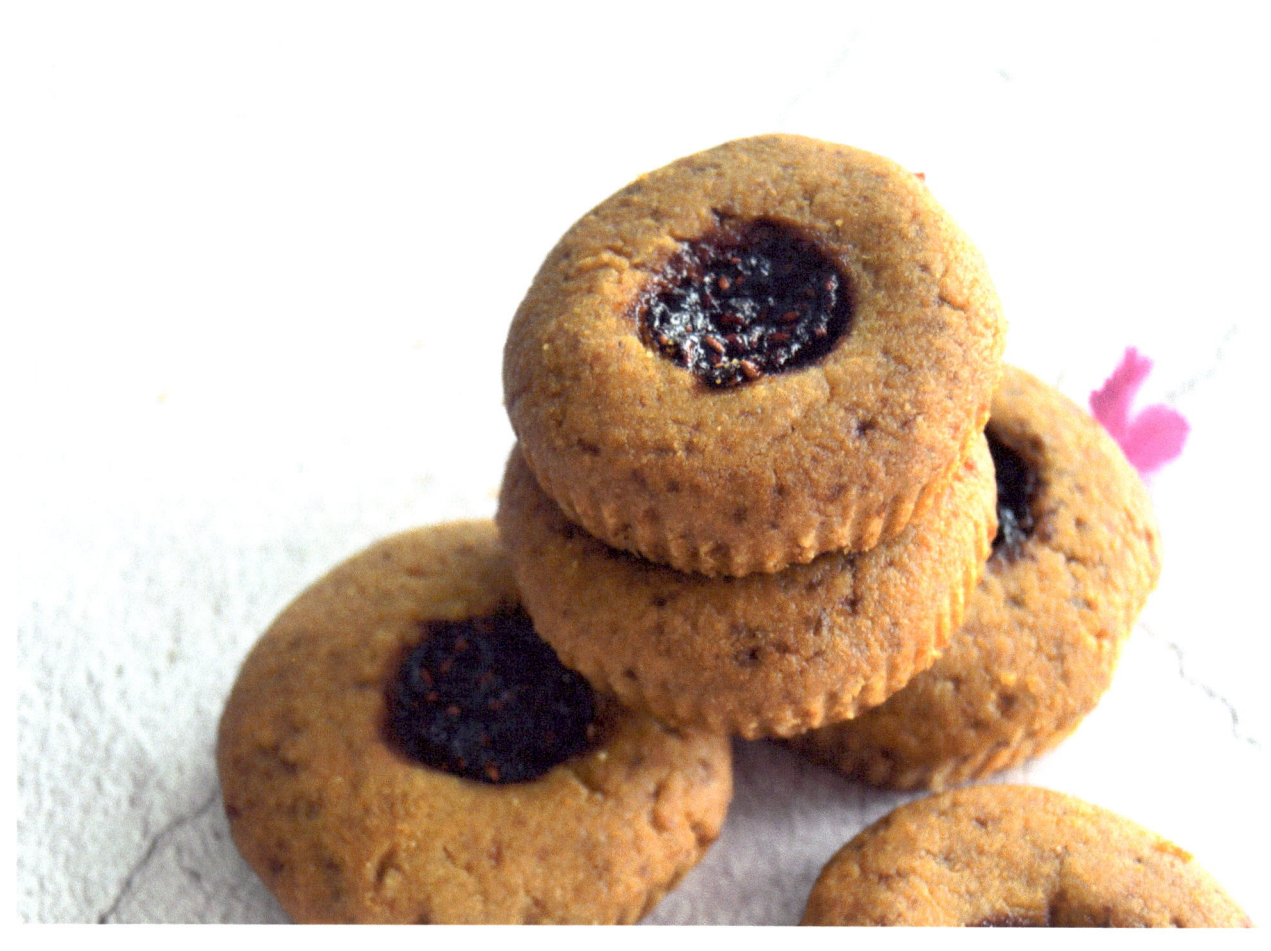

HALLONGROTTOR
SWEDISH STYLE RASPBERRY CAVES

Time - 1 hour
Serves - 18-20 pieces

Ingredients
175 g vegan butter or coconut oil
220 g whole wheat flour or almond flour
1 tsp baking powder
1 tsp vanilla extract
100 g coconut sugar
1/4 cup raspberry jam

1. Pre-heat oven to 200° C.
In a bowl, mix vegan butter, coconut sugar, vanilla and baking powder together until fluffy.

2. Then add the flour and mix thoroughly with your hands until combined. Place 20 mini cupcake mould on a baking sheet.

3. Then divide the dough into 17-18 pieces and roll them into little balls.

4. Place the balls in the cupcake forms and gently press a little hole with your finger in the middle of each ball.

5. Then place about 1-2 tsp raspberry jam in each of the holes.

6. Bake for about 18-20 minutes.

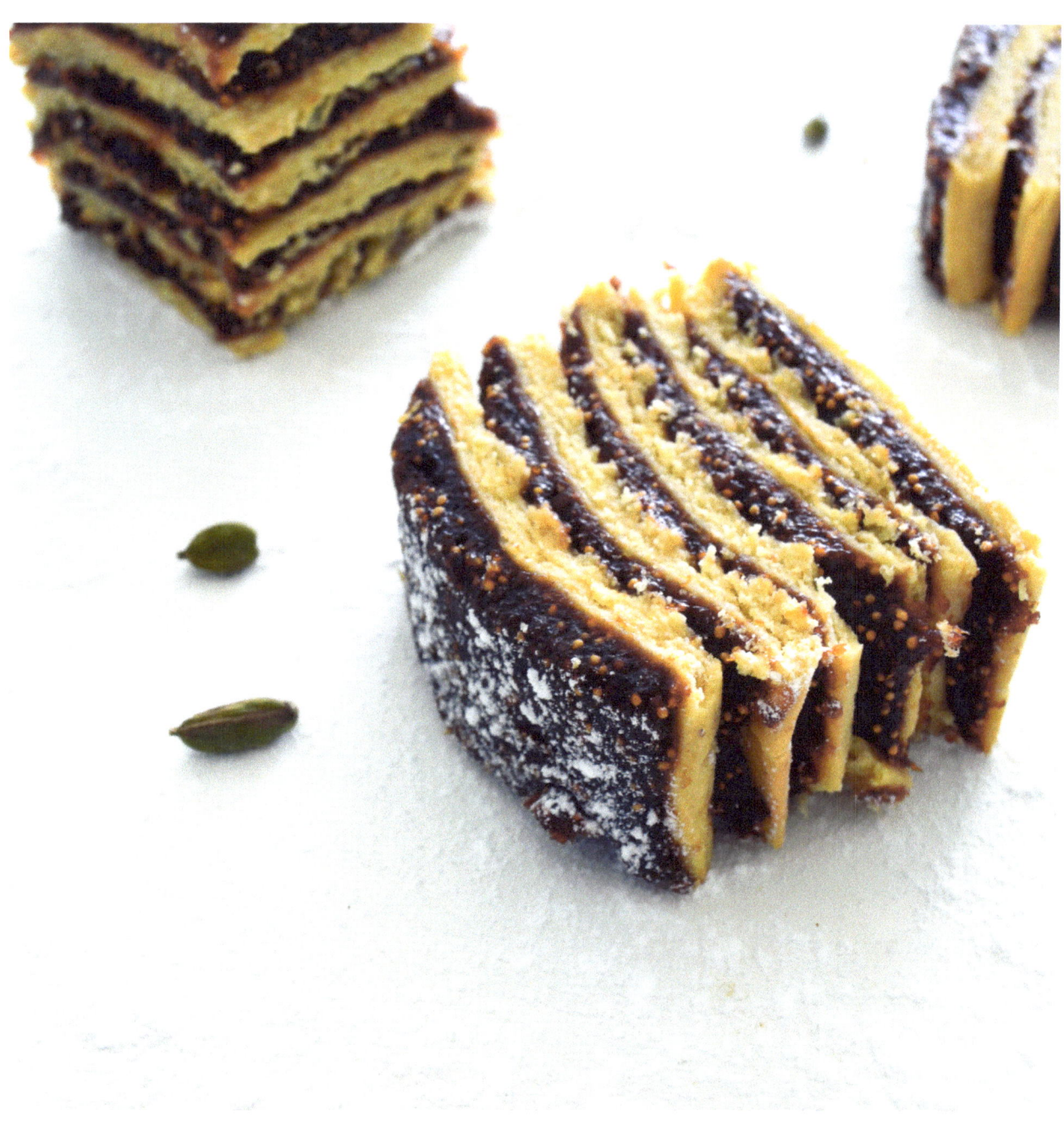

ICELANDIC VINARTERTA

Time - 1 hour
Serves - 6-8

Dough

150 g vegan butter
40 g confectionery sugar
4 tbsp lupin powder or ground flax
+ 100 ml water
1/2 tsp ground cardamom
1 tsp baking powder
1 tsp vanilla extract
2 tbsp almond milk

Filling

1 cup water
500 g dried figs
1 lemon juice
1 tsp cardamom
1 tbsp vodka
1 tsp vanilla extract
30 g coconut sugar
1/2 tsp cinnamon

1. Place dried figs into the pot, cover with 1 cup water. Bring to boil until absorb all the water content. Place them into the food processor, add the rest of filling ingredients; lemon juice, 1 tbsp cardamom, vanilla extract, coconut sugar and cinnamon. Mix on high speed until combined well. Transfer mixture in a bowl. Set aside.
2. Pre-heat oven to 180° C.
3. In a medium bowl, mix 4 tsp egg replacer (lupin or flax) and 100 ml. warm water. Add the butter, sugar, vanilla extract and mix together until combined well. Place mixture into the food processor, add flour, cardamom and baking powder. Mix on high speed until get dough.
4. Remove dough from the food processor. Divide into 7 pieces. Roll dough out on to a floured surface using a rolling pin, give a thing and long shape.
5. Place a baking sheet in a 12 inch cake pan. Place dough in to the pan. Bake for 10 min until soft, but not browned. When the layers are soften, you can easily cut them. When it is baked, let cool it for 5 min at least. Using a knife, spread a layer of the fig mixture over the crust. Place the second crust layer over top. 6. Spread the fig mixture again. Repeat the same process for remaining 5 pieces.
7. Slice it. Keep it in a cool and dry place up to 3 days. Decorate with confectionery sugar if desired.

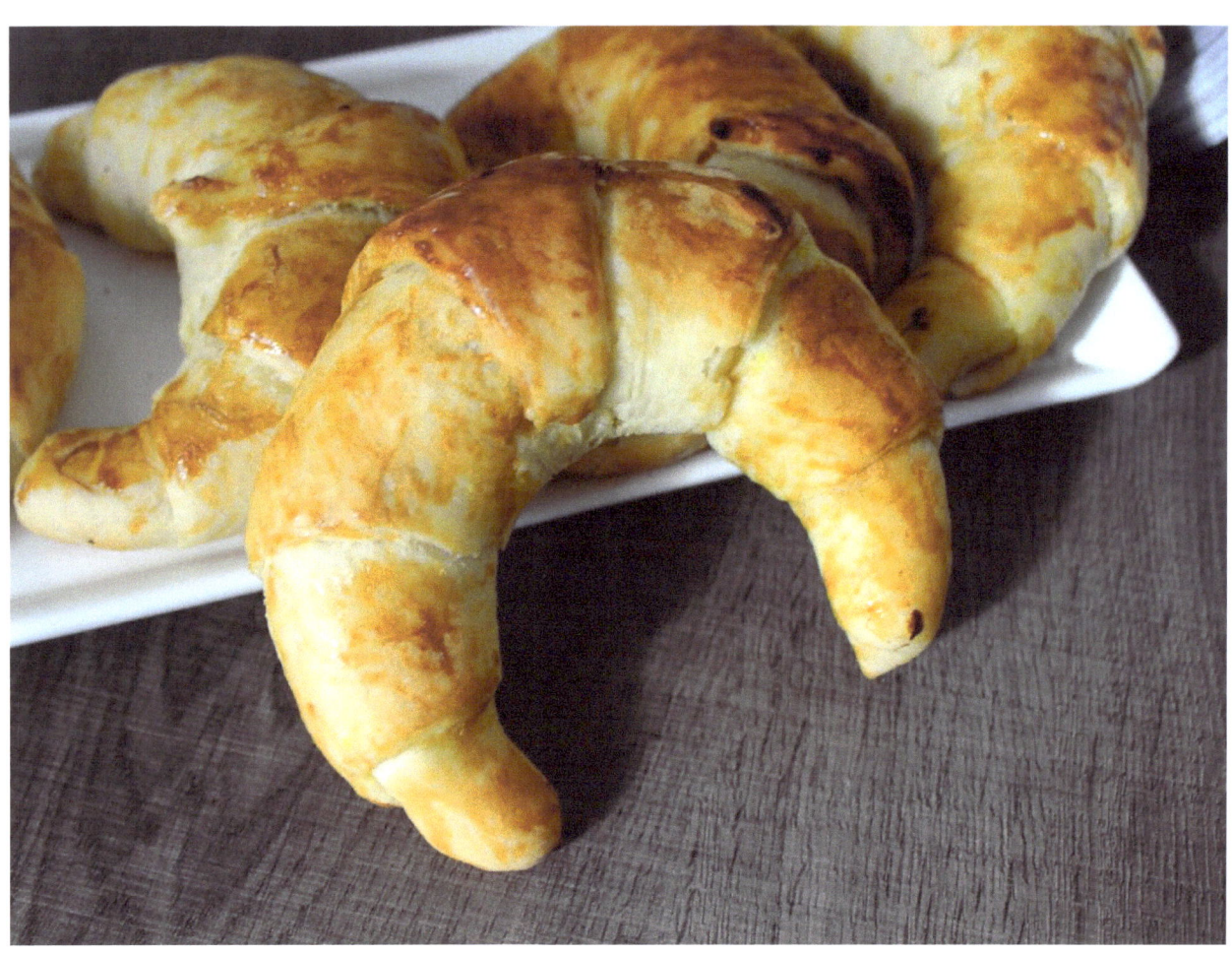

CROISSANT

Time - 2 hrs
Serves - 6-8

Ingredients
1 + 1/2 tbsp active dry yeast
1 tbsp coconut sugar
400 ml water
2 tsp salt
550 g 11%-12% protein all-purpose type of flour or if you can find it a finer ground 00 flour in that same protein range
2 tbsp olive oil
280 g vegan butter
1-2 tbsp carob molasses + 4-8 tbsp water for brushing

1. In a large bowl, whisk active dry yeast, water, oil, sugar, flour and salt together. Mix and knead with your hands for about 10 minutes or until get smooth dough. Cover and chill the dough for at least 1 hour.

2. Transfer dough to a floured surface, make 10 small piece from dough, roll each piece widely using a rolling pin. Before putting on top of each other, brush melted vegan butter between each dough piece. Freeze for 15 minutes.

3. When you remove dough from the freezer, roll it widely in to a rectangular or round form.

4. Take remaining vegan butter and spread over the dough. Cut it in to small triangle pieces. Throw a small slit per triangle.

5. Wrap it and give a croissant shape bending their tails.

6. Pre-heat oven to 180° C.

7. In a small bowl, mix 1 tbsp carob molasses and 4 tbsp water. Brush over the croissant. Bake them until they are brown color.

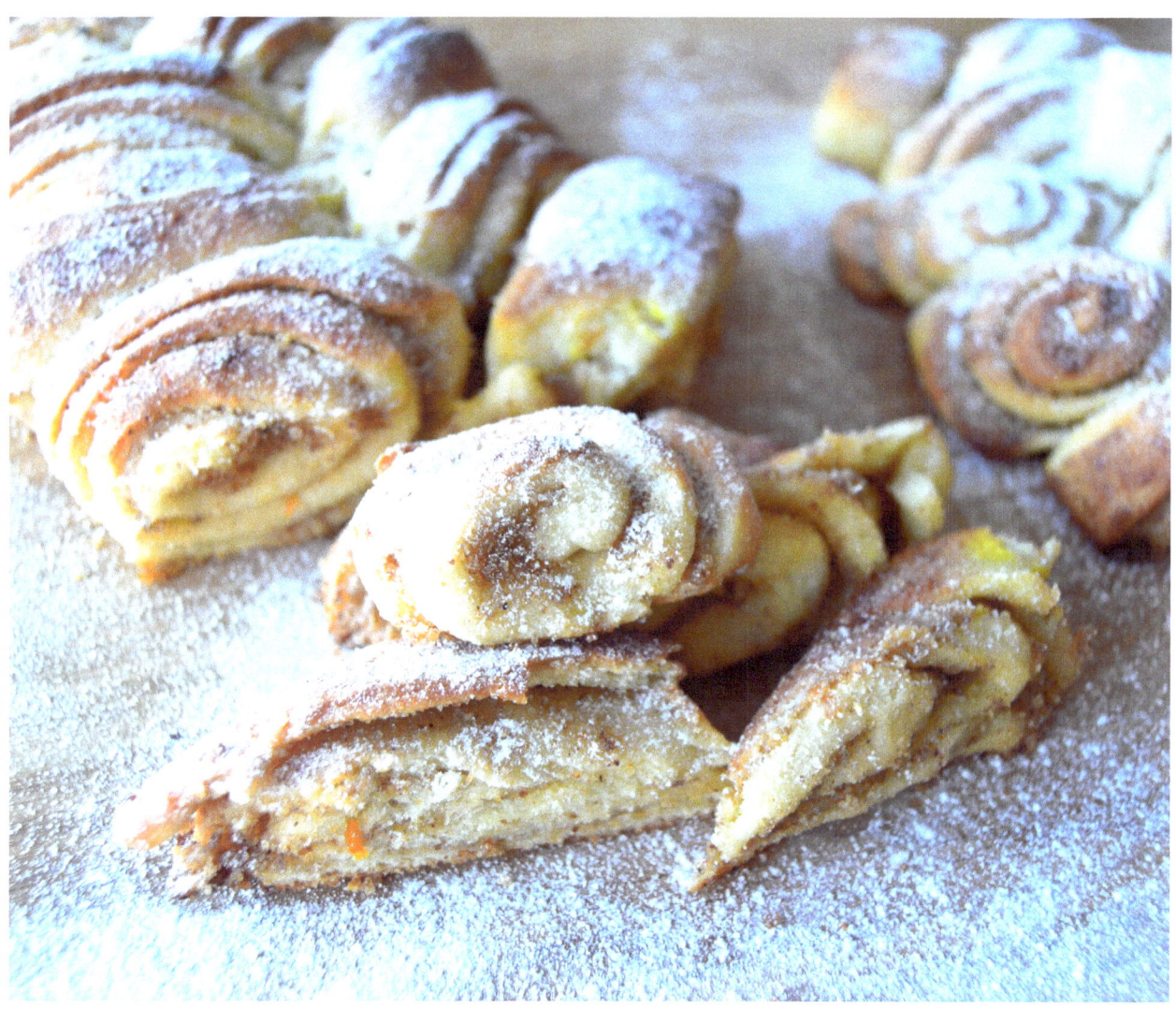

VETELÄNGDER
SWEDISH ALMOND BREAD

Time - 1 hour
Serves - 6-8

Dough
400 g all purpose flour
250 g lukewarm plant milk
8 g dry active yeast
40 g vegan butter
60 g coconut sugar
1 tbsp orange zest
1/4 tsp salt

Filling
1 cup almond flour
1/4 cup coconut sugar
4 tbsp coconut oil
1/2 tsp cinnamon
1/4 tsp cardamom
1 tsp vanilla bean powder
1 tbsp ground flaxseed
3 tbsp water

Toppings
1 tbsp carob molasses
2 tbsp ground flaxseed + 5 tbsp water
2 tbsp confectioners sugar for dusting or coconut flour

1. Mix yeast, lukewarm milk and sugar in a large bowl until yeast is dissolved. Let it rest to activate for 15 minutes. In a small bowl, mix flaxseed and water together. Let it rest in the refrigerator for 15-20 minutes until get sticky.

2. When yeast is activated, then add flour, flax mixture, orange zest, salt mix on low until combined well, then add the vegan butter, mix on medium speed for 5-6 minutes or until come together well.

3. Transfer dough on to the floured surface, knead with your hands for 3-4 minutes. Place dough in a large bowl, cover the bowl with a clean towel. Let it rest in a warm place for 40-45 minutes.

4. When it doubled in size, transfer on to the floured surface, knead for 2-3 minutes. Divide dough into two pieces.
Pre-heat oven to 225° C. In a large bowl, place all filling ingredients and whisk together on high speed for 4-5 minutes. Using a rolling pin roll the dough 20x25 cm rectangle. Spread almond paste over the dough using a silicon spatula. Roll the dough into a tight log. Cut the log in equal pieces with a knife.

4. Repeat the same process for the remaining dough. Place a baking sheet onto the baking pan. Shape the pieces by sticking together right and left. In a small bowl mix egg replacer (flax) and water. Brush the tops of the bread with egg replacer. Bake for 15 minutes until golden browned. Let cool at least 20 minutes. Sprinkle with confectioners sugar. Slice and serve!

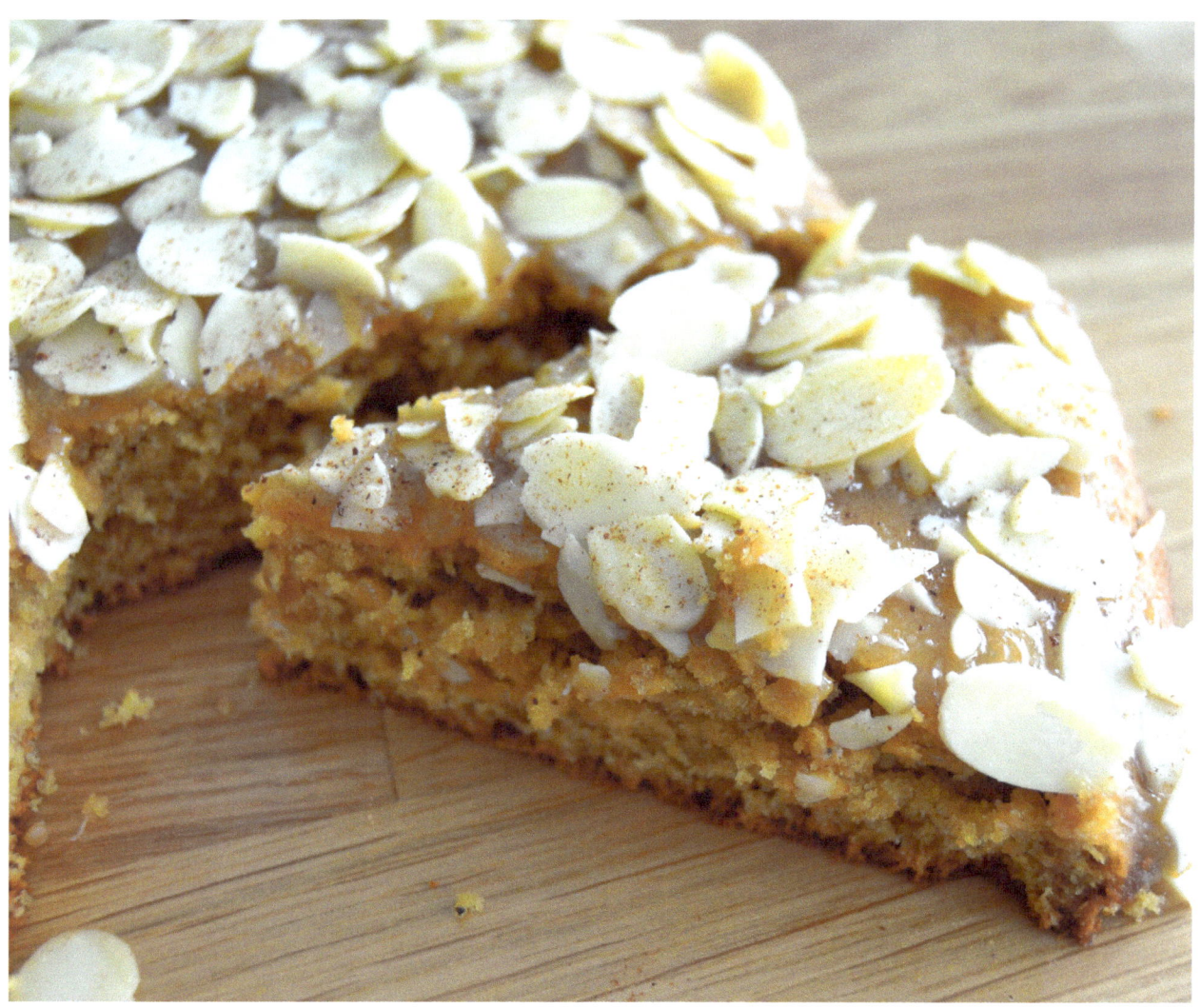

TOSCATÅRTA
SWEDISH ALMOND CAKE

Time - 50 minutes
Serves - 6

Ingredients
2 tsp ground flaxseed + 90 ml water
50 g coconut sugar
2 tsp vanilla extract
4 tbsp maple syrup
50 g coconut oil
175 g all purpose flour
30 g chestnut flour
80 ml almond milk
9 g baking powder

Glaze
50 g vegan butter
80 g sliced almonds
60 g maple syrup
1 tbsp coconut flour
2 tbsp almond meal

1. Pre-heat oven to 200° C. Lightly oil the spring-form pan, set aside.

2. In a large bowl, whisk coconut sugar, maple, ground flaxseed and water until fluffy. Add the coconut oil and mix well together.

3. Then add all purpose flour, chestnut flour, baking powder, vanilla extract and almond milk. Using a mixer, whisk on high speed for 5-6 minutes

4. Pour mixture in a grassed spring-form pan.

5. Bake at the bottom of the oven for 20-25 minutes or until golden browned. When it is baked, remove from the oven and set aside. Let it cool while making glazing sauce.

6. To make glazing, mix all the ingredients except sliced almonds in a bowl. Then pour over the cake. Decorate with sliced almonds. Let it sit in the fridge for 1 hour. Then slice and serve.

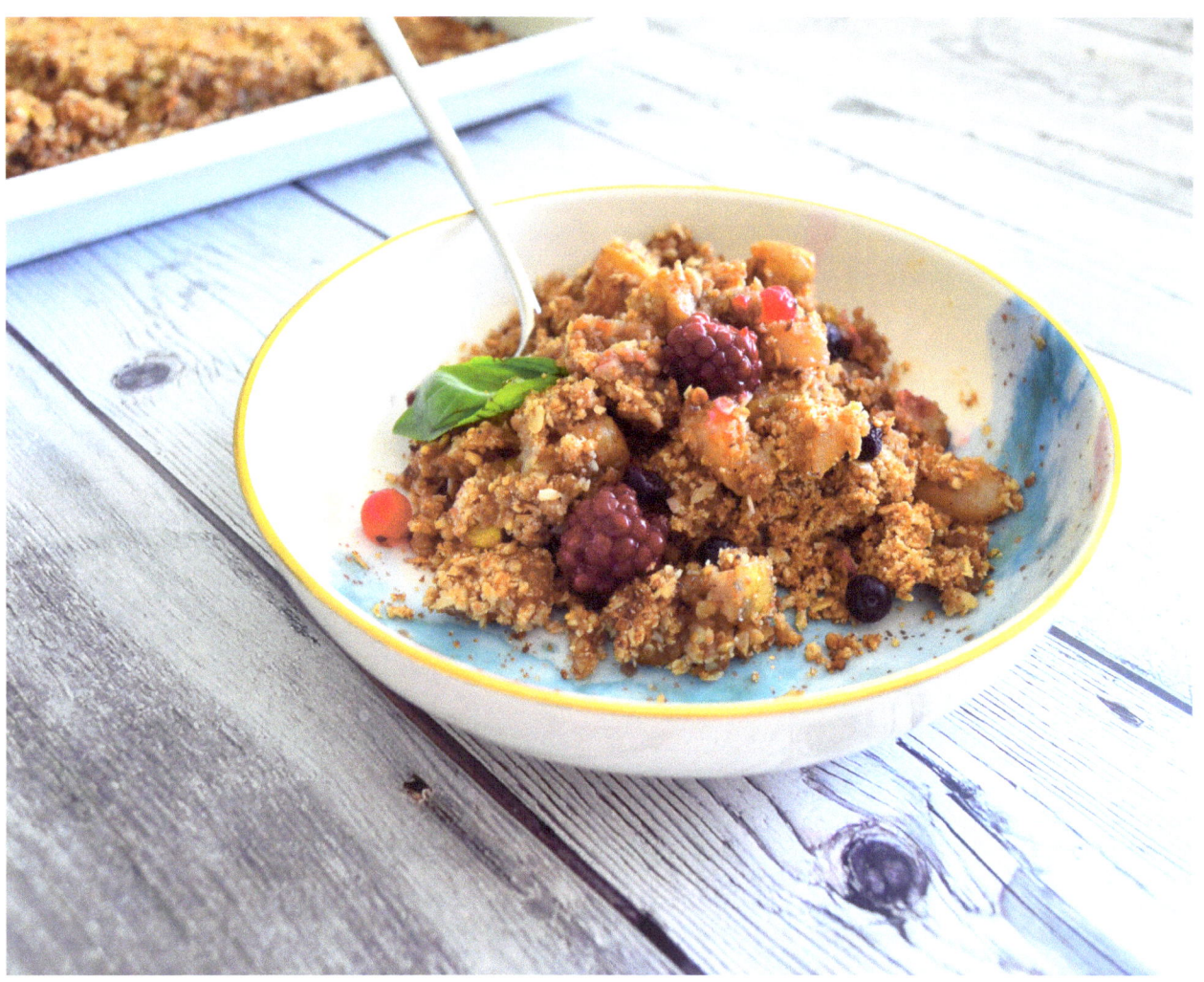

PEAR WALNUT CRUMBLE

Time - 50 minutes
Serves - 4-5

Ingredients
1 + 1/2 cup rolled oats
1 cup crushed walnuts
1/2 tsp salt
7-8 tbsp coconut sugar
3 pears cubed
1 tsp cinnamon
1 tsp cardamom
1 tsp vanilla extract
3 tbsp lemon juice
1 tsp tapioca
3 tbsp almond meal
1 tbsp coconut oil

1. Preheat oven to 180° C.
Place a parchment paper onto the baking pan.

2. Place pear cubes into the bowl, add 3 tbsp sugar, cinnamon, cardamom, 1/4 tsp salt, vanilla extract, lemon juice and tapioca, toss together. Cover with foil and bake for about 15 minutes. Set aside.

3. Place 1 cup rolled oats, walnuts, 1/4 tsp salt, vanilla, 2 tbsp coconut sugar and vegan butter into the food processor, mix on high speed. Transfer mixture into the baking pan. Press down into an even layer with your hands. Open foil and spread pear mixture over the crust layer.

4. Place 2 tablespoon coconut sugar, almond flour, 1/2 cup rolled oats and 1 tablespoon coconut oil into the food processor, mix on high speed and make crumble with your hands.

5. Top with crumble topping.

6. Place pan into the oven. Bake for 20-25 minutes or until golden browned.

7. Serve with whipped coconut cream and your favorite berries or icecream if desired.

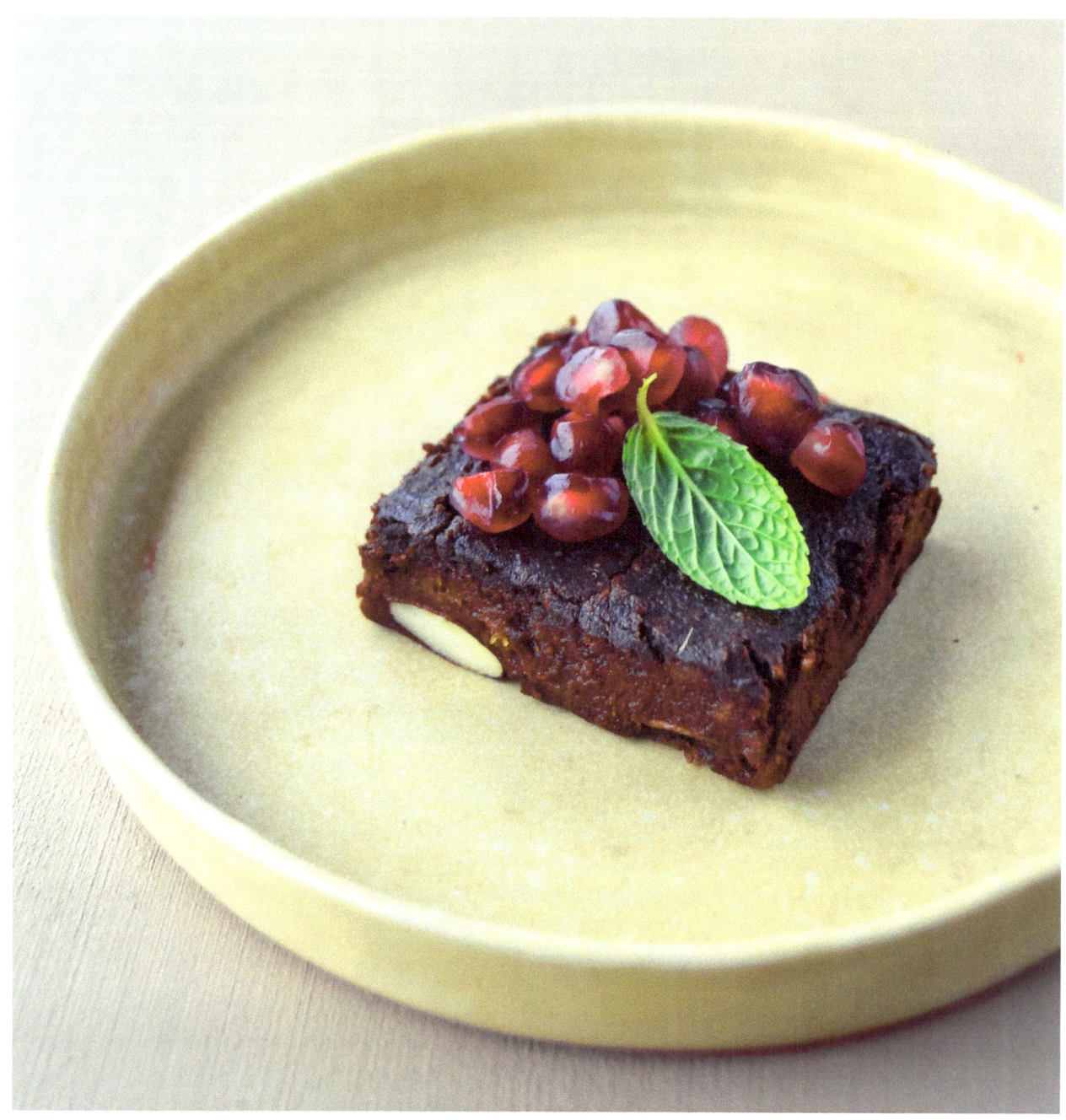

SWEET POTATO CHOCOLATE CAKE

Time - 40 minutes
Serves - 4-6

Ingredients
265 g sweet potato cooked
60 g almond butter
30 g gluten free oat flour
5 tbsp cacao
5 tbsp maple syrup
1/2 tsp baking powder
1/4 tsp salt

1. Place cooked sweet potato in a bowl, mash using a fork.
2. Then add the rest of the ingredients over the mashed potato.
3. Mix well until well combined.
4. Preheat oven to 185° C.
5. Place the mixture in a square pan / pyrex with parchment paper.
6. Bake at 185° C for 25-30 minutes.
7. Remove from the oven, let it cool for 15-20 minutes.
8. Serve with pomegranates or bananas and sour forest fruits of your choice.

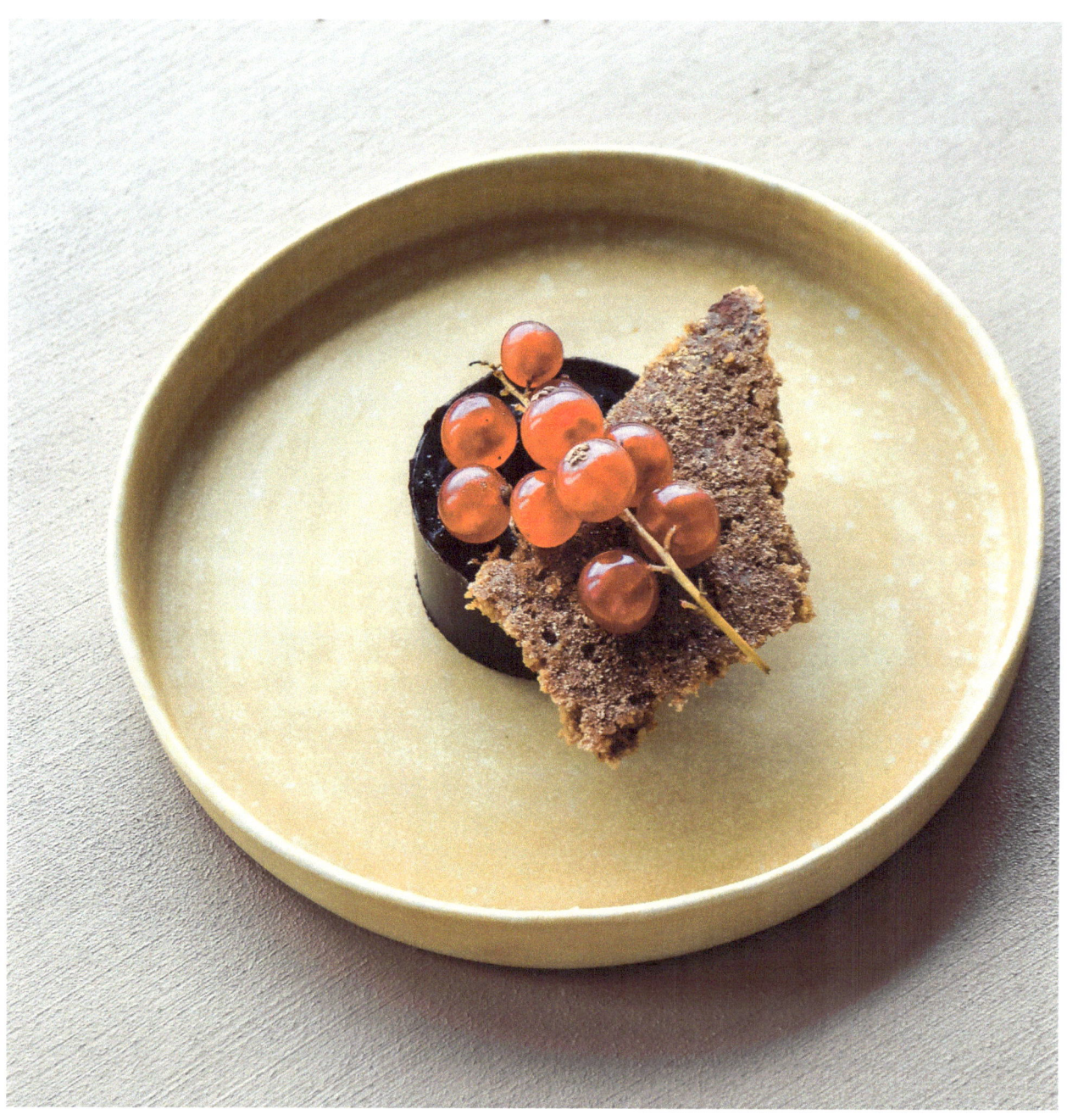

CHOCOLATE MOUSSE WITH ALMOND BRITTLE

Mousse
100 g vegan 60% dark chocolate
270 g cashew milk
1 tsp (2 g) agar agar

Brittle
100 g almond flour
3 tbsp maple syrup
A pinch salt

1. To make brittle, preheat the oven to 150° C.

2. Gently mix the almond flour with the agave syrup until it feels like marzipan.

3. Between two pieces of baking paper, roll out the dough to as thin as possible (1 mm).
Take off the top paper and bake for 7-8 minutes, until golden.
Keep in a dry place until needed.

4. To make mousse, mix the agar agar and milk together in a pot. Over low heat, bring to a rolling boil.

5. Put the chocolate in a bowl. In three or four additions, mixing after each, pour the hot milk and agar agar over the chocolate.

6. Blend until the mixture looks shiny and very elastic.

7. Pour in moulds and let it sit at least 30 minutes before serving.

8. Serve with brittle and forest fruits at room temperature.

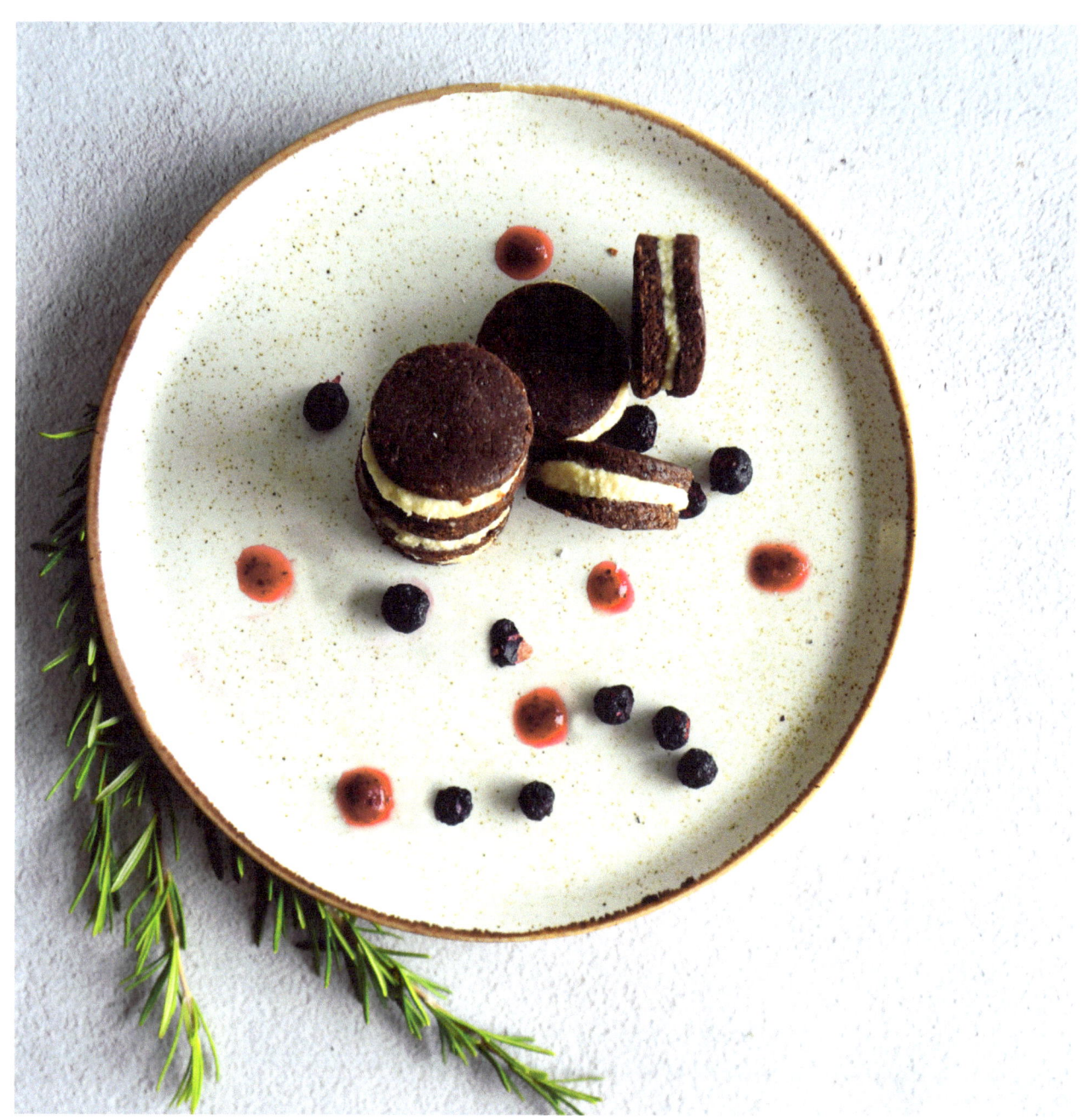

RAW OREOS

Time - 50 minutes
Serves - 6-8

Cookie
1/2 cup oat flour,
1/2 cup coconut flour
2 tbsp cacao powder,
8-10 large medjool dates pitted, soaked in hot water,
1 tbsp melted coconut oil
1-2 tbsp water

Filling
1/2 cup raw cashews soaked
2 tbsp cacao butter melted
2 tbsp lemon juice
1-2 tbsp plant milk
2 tbsp maple
1/2 tsp vanilla extract

1. Place all dough ingredients into food processor and mix until it reaches a dough-like consistency.

2. Line a flat surface or large cutting board with parchment paper and place the dough in the center. Use a rolling pin to roll the dough into an even, roughly 1/4-inch-thick rectangle. Cut in circle shapes with cookie cutter.

3. Place all the filling ingredients into a blender, mix on high speed until you get paste form. Top half of the cookies with roughly 1 tsp filling cream.

4. Put in the freezer to chill for just a few minutes. Then put another circle top on the cookie.

5. Refrigerate at least 2 hours before consuming.
They tend to soften when at room temperature so keep them in the fridge.
You can also keep them in the freezer up to 1 month.

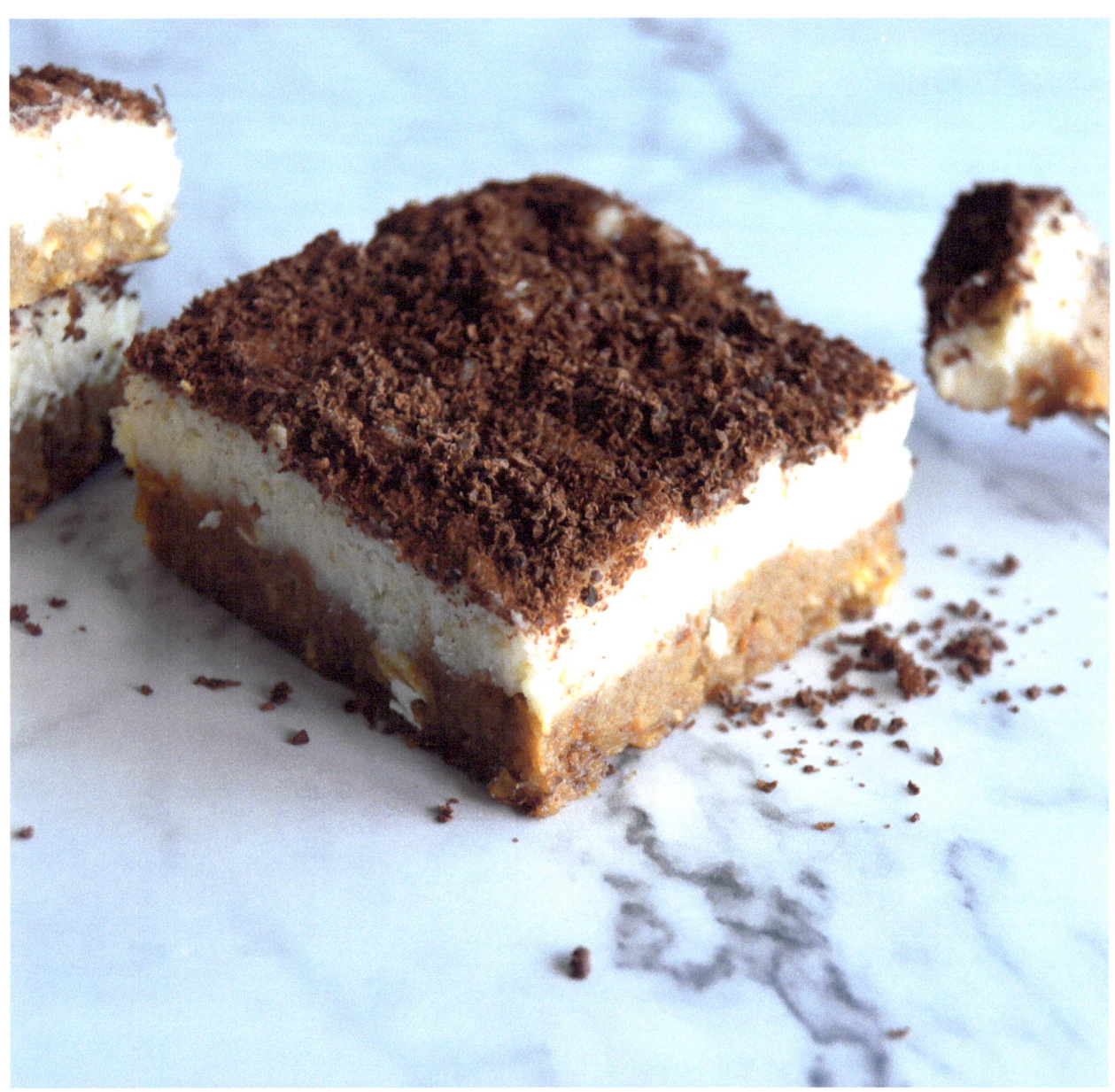

RAW COFFEE CAKE

Crust

1/2 cup almond flour
2 tbsp rolled oats
1 tbsp activated dehydrated buckini
60 g raw cashews
2 tbsp coconut oil
6 large medjool dates
3 tbsp espresso
A pinch salt

Cream Layer

100 g raw cashews soaked and drained
40 g cacao butter melted
2 tbsp maple
2 tbsp coconut oil
3 tbsp coconut butter melted
7 tbsp cashew milk

1. Process all crust layer ingredients in your food processor until sticky.

2. Press the mixture into a 15 cm cake tin and place in the freezer to set while you are making the cream layer..

3. Add all the cream layer ingredients in the blender. Blend until smooth.

4. Pour mixture over the cake. Freeze for 2 hours before serving.

5. Before serving, top with shredded vegan chocolate or dust raw cacao if desired.

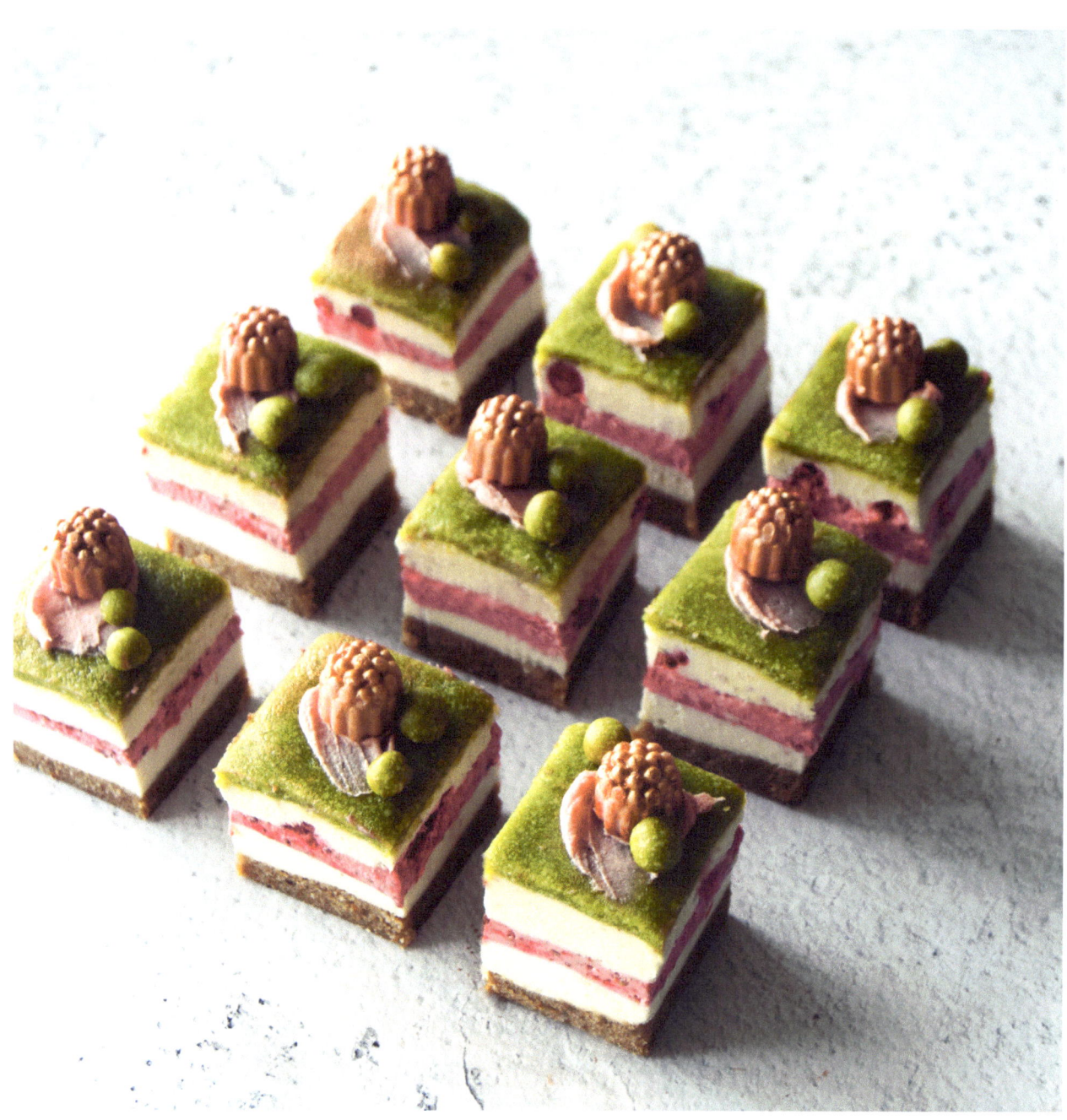

RAW SWEDISH PRINCESS CAKE

Time - 2 hrs
Serves - 9

Base
90 g almonds
100 g date paste
35 g coconut flour
1 tbsp coconut oil
1/2 tsp vanilla powder

Filling
160 g raw cashews soaked
3 tbsp maple syrup
3 tbsp lemon juice
40 g coconut oil melted
25 g cacao butter melted
100 g coconut cream

Mid Layer
150 g raspberry chia jam
115 g filling cream
15 g cacao butter

Green Marzipan
1/2 tsp matcha powder
90 g raw almond flour
4 tbsp maple syrup
20 g raw coconut flour
1/4 tsp bitter almond extract

1. To make the base add the almonds and to a food processor and blitz until they are finely ground. Add the remaining ingredients for the base and continue to blitz until all the ingredients are broken down into a crumb. The mixture should press together like a dough between your fingers. Press the dough into the bottom of your cake tin. Pack it down firmly and set aside while you making filling.
2. To prepare the filling, add the cashews, coconut cream, maple syrup, lemon juice to your blender. Blend until they are smooth. Lastly add in the melted coconut oil, and coconut butter then blend further for 30 seconds to incorporate the oil into the mixture. Take around 100 gr of the cream and set aside to use it in mid layer later. Pour half of the remaining cream over the cake crust. Place in the freezer to set for 20 minutes to set in order to prevent mixed layers.
3. Make raspberry chia jam according to raw jam recipe in this book. Place in a bowl, add 100 gr of the filling cream and melted cacao butter. Mix well in the bowl. Set aside.
4. Place almond and coconut flour into food processor, combine well. Then add agave syrup, almond extract and matcha. Mix until you get sticky dough. If it is too wet, then add more almond flour.
5. When first cream layer is done, remove from the freeezer, add raspberry layer over the cashew filling, then set in the freezer next 25 minutes. Then pour remaining cashew filling. Freeze for 45 minutes. Remove cake from the mold. Cover with princess layer (green marzipan. Keep in the refrigerator for next 30 minutes before cutting and serve.

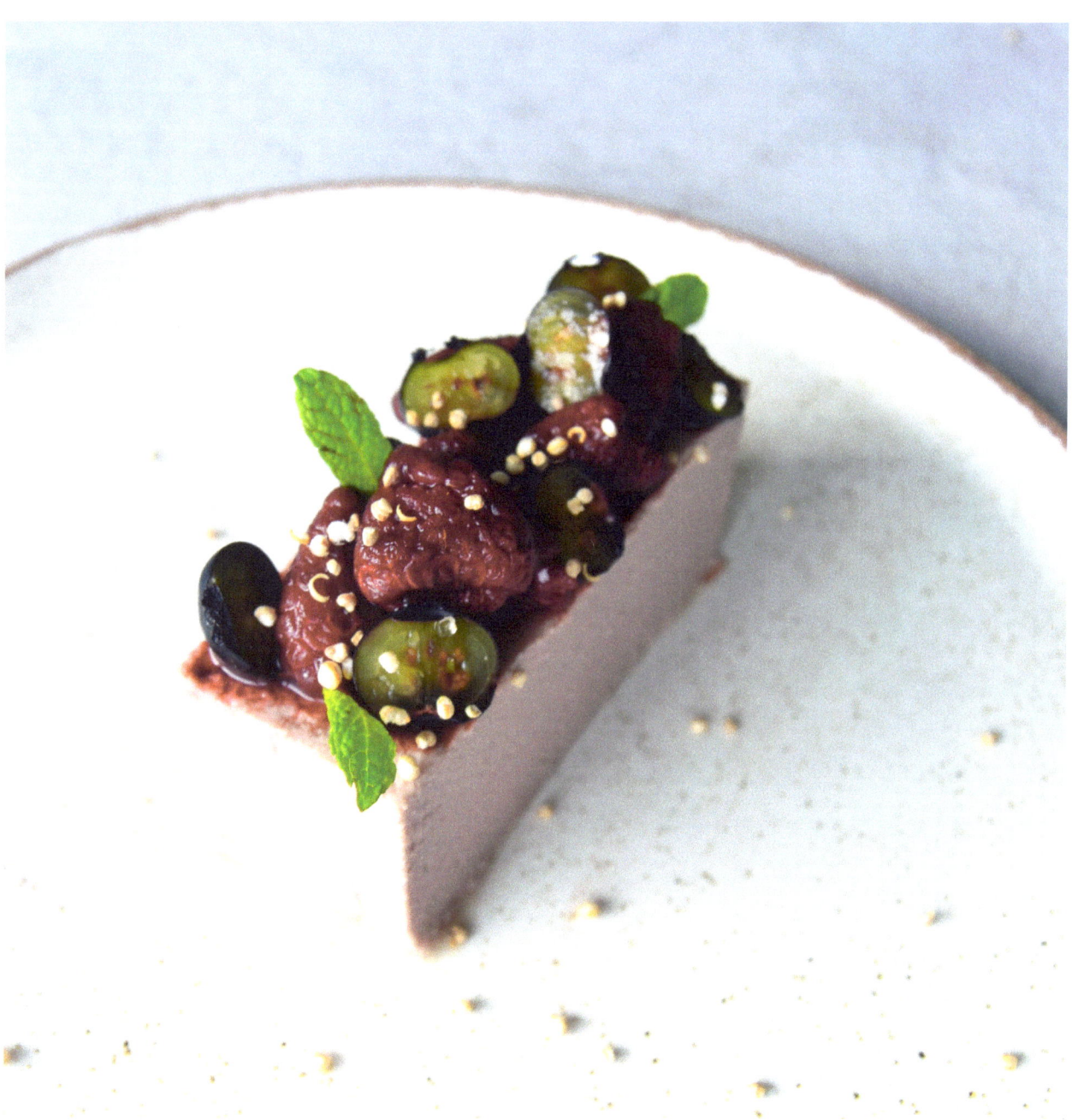

RASPBERRY PANNA COTTA

Time - 30 minutes
Serves - 2

Ingredients
1 can full-fat coconut milk
1/2 cup fresh raspberries
3/4 tsp agar agar powder
1/4 cup coconut sugar

Raspberry Sauce
1 cup fresh raspberries
1 + 1/2 tsp coconut sugar

Raspberries and halved blueberries for garnish
Fresh mint for garnish
Popped quinoa for garnish

1. Add 1/2 cup of raspberries together with the coconut milk in a blender and blend until smooth. Place a nut milk bag over a pot and pour in the raspberry-coconut mixture, squeeze to remove the harder bits of the raspberries.

2. Whisk in the agar powder and sugar and bring it to a boil. Let it simmer for 2-3 minutes, then fill the mixture into small glass or porcelain containers.
Let them sit in the fridge overnight.

3. For the raspberry sauce simply simmer the defrosted raspberries together with the sugar in a small pot and mash the raspberries a bit.

4. To serve, go around the edges of the panna cotta with a knife until you can take it out of the form. Top with the warm raspberry sauce.

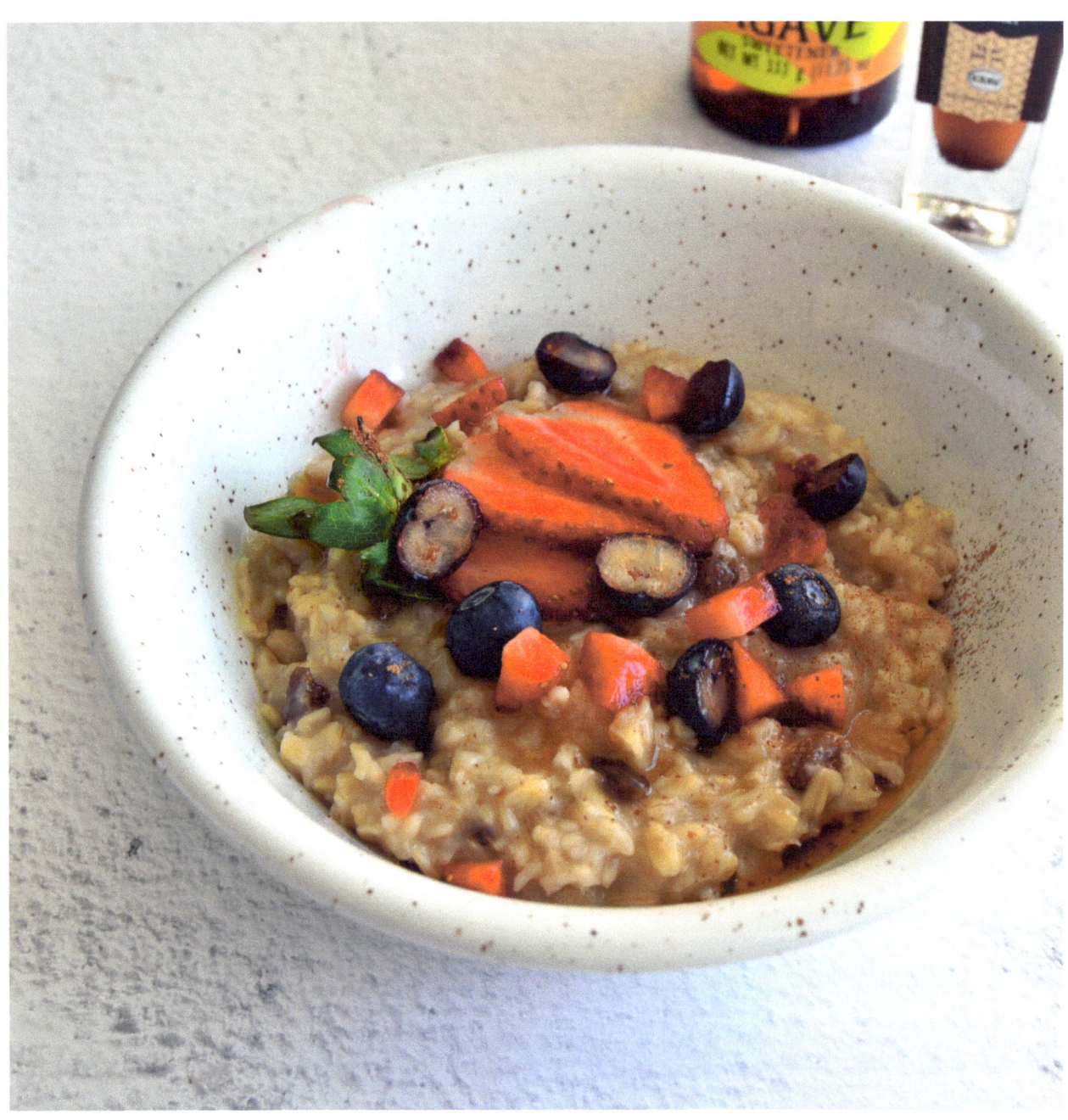

OATMEAL

Time - 20 minutes
Serves - 2

Ingredients
1 cup rolled oats
1.5 -2 cups water or almond milk
1 tbsp maple or more if you need
(alternatively dates can be added)
1/4 tsp pink himalayan salt
1/2 tsp cinnamon extract or powder

Toppings
Buckini (activated & dehydrated buckwheats)
Sliced strawberries and blueberries
or whatever you like.

1. Soak the oats for at least a couple of hours minimum, but better to soak them overnight in 4 cups of water if you have the time. In the morning strain and add 2 cups of clear water or plant-based milk.

2. If you're using dates in the place of maple , you may want to soak the dates as well, you can use the date soak water as part, or all, of the 2 cups needed in the recipe to make it just a little bit sweeter.

3. Next ,place the rinsed oats, dates, and the two cups of water (or, use some of the date soak water) in a blender or food processor and blend or process on high speed for about 25 seconds or until the mixture is smooth.

4. To make RAW, place into a bowl and cover. Move to food dehydrator. Cook at 42° C for 2-3 hours or until soften and warm enough. Mix well. Taste it, add more cinnamon or sweetener if you need.
To cooked version, transfer mixture in a pot, on low-medium heat stir well until soften enough. Once cooked, divide between bowls.
5. Top with chopped blueberries, strawberries, cinnamon powder and buckinis. Drizzle extra maple or agave syrup if desired.

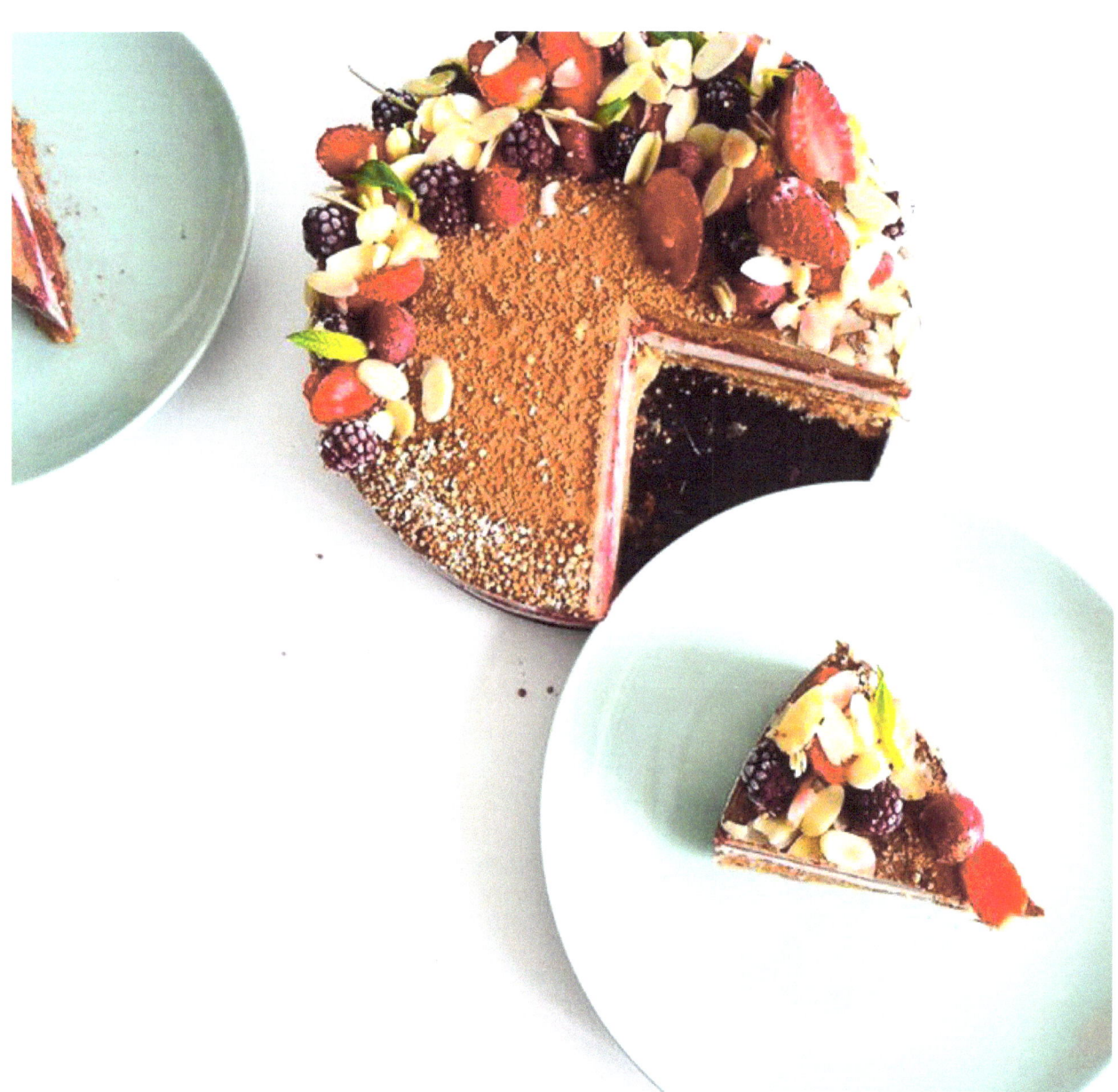

4 LAYER RAW CAKE WITH FOREST FRUITS

Time - 2 hrs
Serves - 8

Crust
140 g peanut flour
100 g almond flour
2 tbsp desiccated coconut
280 gr. medjool dates

2nd Layer
220 g pre-soaked raw cashews
2 tbsp organic cold press coconut oil
3 tbsp raw cacao butter melted
2 tbsp maple syrup
3 tbsp lemon juice
2 tsp vanilla extract
80 g banana

Third Layer
220 g pre-soaked raw cashews
3 tbsp lingonberry powder
2 tbsp agave syrup
2 tbsp lemon juice
2 tbsp cold press coconut oil
2 tbsp raw cacao butter melted or irish moss

Top Layer
2 ripe avocado
4 tbsp agave syrup
1 tbsp lemon juice
2 tbsp raw cacao butter melted
1 tbsp coconut oil
1 tbsp raw cacao powder
1/4 tsp bitter almond extract

1. Place all crust ingredients into the food processor, mix on high speed until completely smooth. Transfer mixture into the springform pan (22 cm). Press with your hands, flatten out. Place into the freezer while making 2nd. layer.

2. Place all 2nd layer ingredients into the blender, mix well until completely smooth. Remove pan from the freezer, pour mixture onto the crust layer. Place it into the freezer again at least 45 minutes.

3. Place all third layer into the blender, mix on high speed until completely smooth. Pour mixture over the 2nd layer. Place into the freezer for 2 hours.

4. Place all top layer ingredients into the food processor, mix well until creamy. Using a double boiler, melt mixture very slowly at 42° C. Pour mixture onto the third layer.

5. Decorate with berries and sliced almonds or your favorite nuts and berries! Let it rest in the freezer for 3-4 hours before cutting.

BLUEBERRY COCONUT CHOCOLATE CAKE

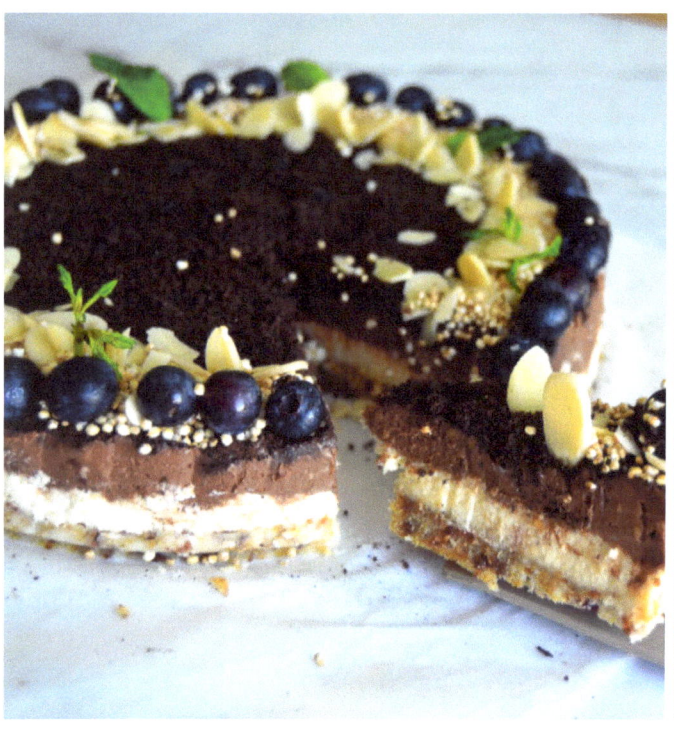
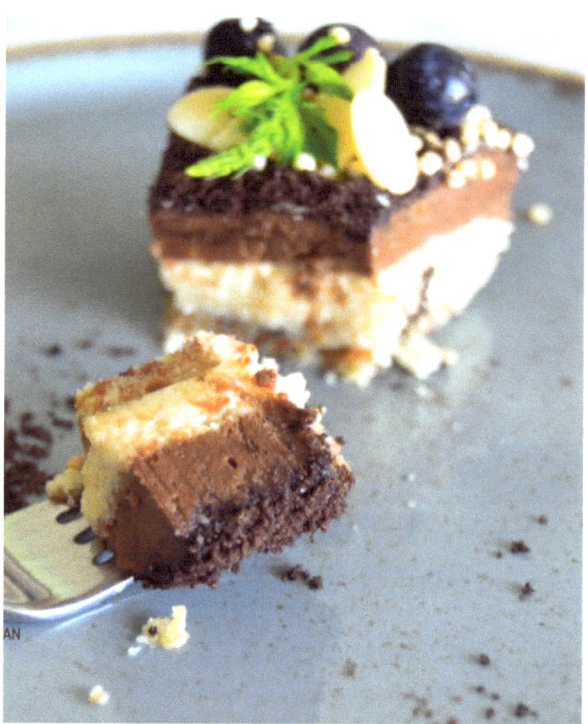

Time - 1 hour
Serves - 8

Crust
170 g medjool dates
150 g almond meal
2 tbsp coconut oil
1/4 tsp salt

White Layer
100 g coconut cream
130 g cashews soaked
2 tbsp maple syrup
1 tsp vanilla bean powder
3 tbsp lemon juice
2 tbsp coconut oil
1 tbsp raw cacao butter melted

Chocolate Layer
260 ripe avocado
2 tbsp lemon juice
180 g raw dark chocolate

Decoration
Raw cacao or shredded chocolate
sliced almonds, quinoa pops or activated dehydrated buckwheats
1 cup fresh blueberries
fresh mint leaves

1. Place all crust ingredients into the food processor, mix on high speed until get dough.

2. Line a parchment paper into the spring-form pan (20 cm). Transfer mixture into the spring-form pan. Press with your hands, flatten out.

3. Place all white layer ingredients into the blender, mix on high speed until get silky and smooth mixture. Pour mixture onto the crust layer. Flatten out using a spatula. Place it into the freezer while preparing chocolate layer.

4. Using a double boiler, melt your chocolate gently.

5. Place the melted chocolate into the blender, add the peeled and pitted avocado and lemon juice. Mix on high speed until get silky mixture.

6. Pour mixture onto the white layer.

7. Sprinkle with shredded chocolate or raw cacao. Decorate with almond slices, quinoa pops and mint leaves. Let it cool in the refrigerator at least 4 hours before serving!

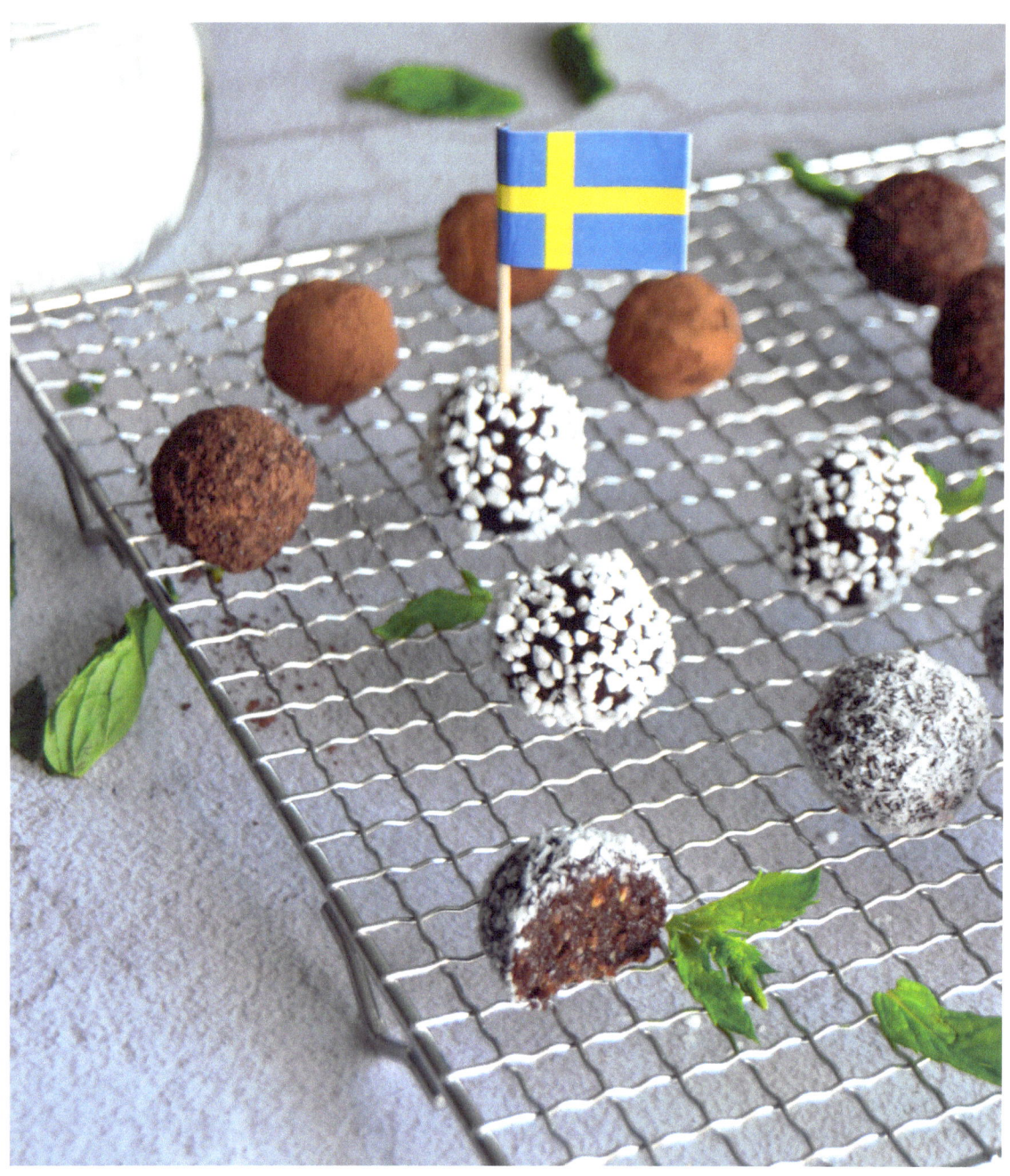

CHOKLADBOLLAR
SWEDISH CHOCOLATE BALLS

Time - 20 minutes
Serves - 8-10

Ingredients
100 g rolled oats
50 g almond flour
130 g soft medjool dates
4 tbsp raw cacao
1/2 tsp vanilla bean powder
2 tbsp maple syrup
5 tbsp espresso

Coating
Desiccated coconut
Shredded vegan chocolate
Swedish pearl sugar

These chokladbollar require no cooking, only moulding by hand. And the procedure may be modified according to personal preference: while chocolate balls are typically rolled in pearl sugar, desiccated coconut or sprinkles can also be used. This simplicity, this versatility, make the chokladboll a plausible and effortless dessert on those occasions when you think you have no dessert, but would like some.

1. Make 1 cup espresso and set aside. Place all ingredients in a food processor and mix on high until you get a smooth dough.

2. Form the balls and roll them into coconut flakes, shredded chocolate or roll them in whatever you desire.

3. Place in the refrigerator for 1 hour before serving! Serve cold!

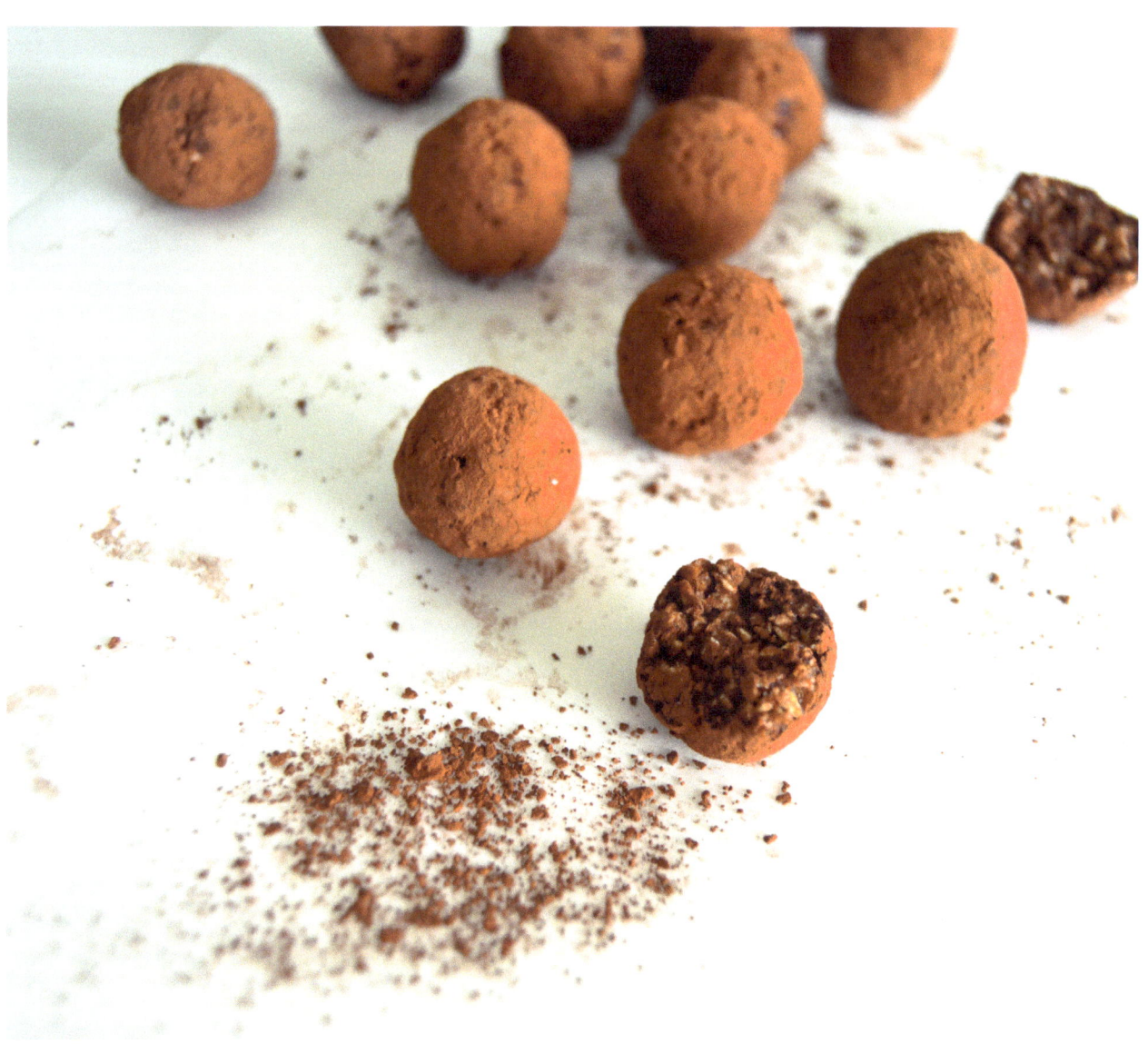

CINNAMON BALLS

Time - 20 minutes
Serves - 12-14

Ingredients
100 g rolled oats
125 g soft medjool dates
1 tbsp raw cacao powder
1 tsp cinnamon
1/2 tsp cardamom
A pinch salt
2 tbsp water or plant-based milk
2 tbsp coconut oil melted

1. Place the rolled oats into the food processor mix on high speed until comes to a crumb form. Then add the dates and mix on high until sticky. (If the dates are not soft, soak beforehand then strain and add to the food processor)

2. Add all the rest of the ingredients and process again, until you get a sticky dough. It should hold together, otherwise add 1-2 tbsp plant-based milk or water.

3. Roll the balls into raw cacao or cinnamon powder according to your choice. Keep in the refrigerator to shape at least one hour, then serve.

AVOCADO CHOCOLATE MOUSSE WITH MULBERRY CRUMBLE

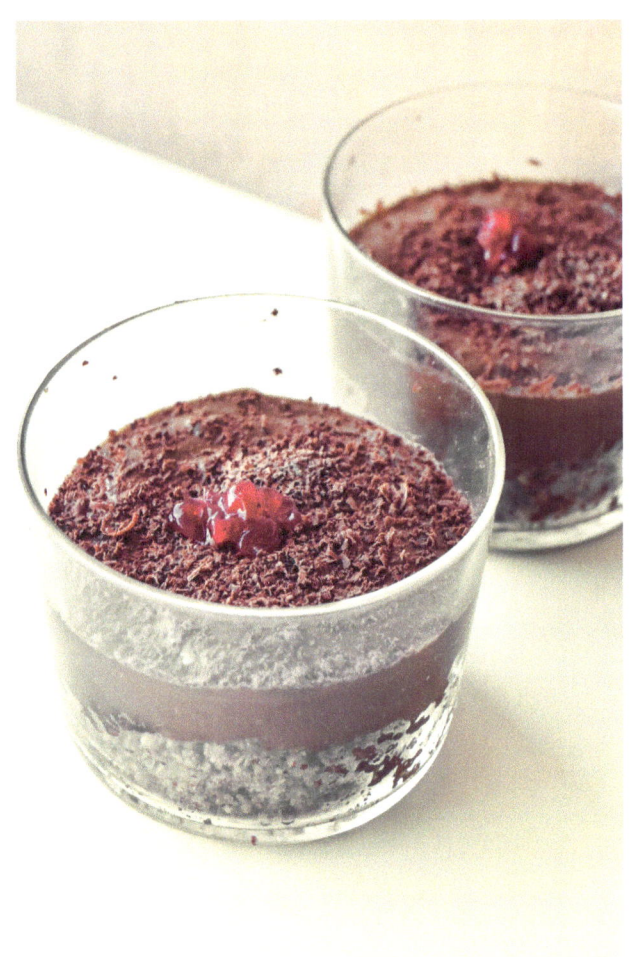
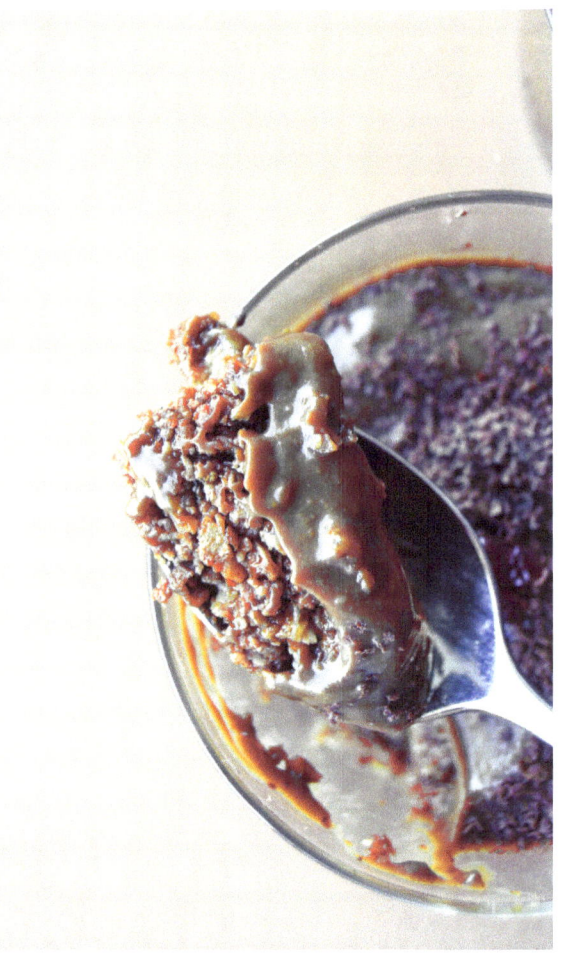

Time - 30 minutes
Serves - 3-4

Crumble
40 g dried white mulberries
40 g hazelnut butter
40 g buckini (activated dehydrated buckwheat groats)
15 g cacao powder
30 g maple syrup
1/8 tsp salt

Mousse
1 ripe avocado (160 g)
30 g raw cacao powder
60 ml maple syrup
60 ml coconut cream (fatty part)
5 drops wild orange essential oil
A pinch salt

1. Throw the white dried mulberry into the food processor and mix it until it comes to a crumb form.
2. Then add the buckinis (buckwheat groats that you soaked in water for 1 hour, rinsed and dehydrated at 46° C for 4-5 hours, beforehand) Mix mulberry and buckini together.
3. Then run the food processor again, adding raw cacao powder, maple syrup, hazelnut butter and salt. Mix in the food processor until everyting combines together.
4. Remove the dough from the food processor and divide between 3-4 mousse jars.
5. Transfer all cream ingredients to a blender. Blend until it becomes a smooth liquid. Taste the mixture, adding a little salt or sweetener if needed. Depending on the variety, softness and fat content of your avocado, you may want to add another tablespoon or two of coconut milk. The consistency should be slightly thick but at the same time pourable fluidity.
6. Pour the mixture on the crumble, gently shake the jars from side to side to prevent bubbles.
7. After 3 hours in the refrigerator it will be ready to serve. Sprinkle some shredded chocolate and top with forest fruits if desired.

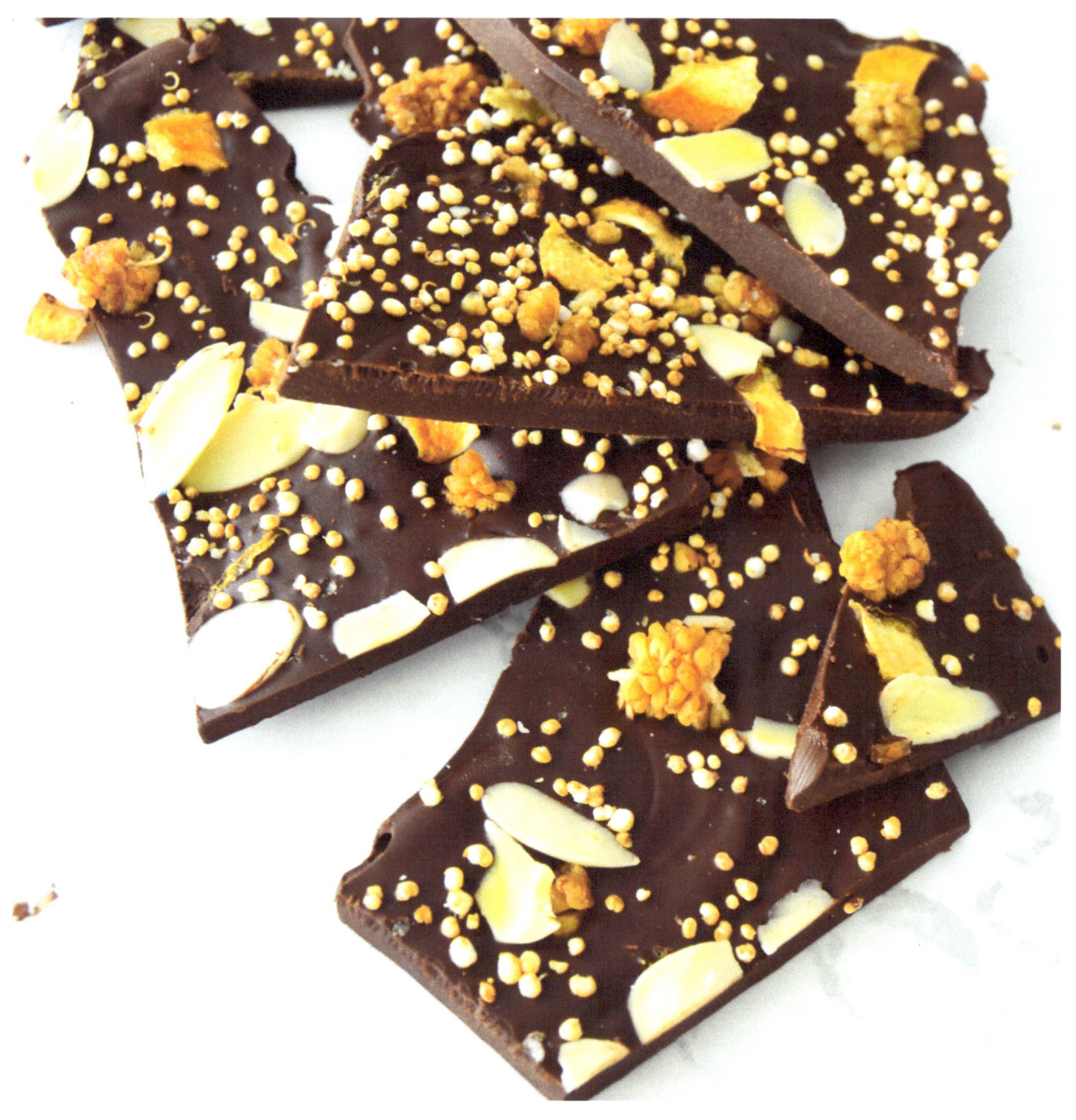

RAW CHOCOLATE

Time - 25 minutes
Serves - 4

Ingredients
60 g raw cacao butter melted
50 g raw coconut oil melted
1 tsp vanilla extract
A handful of crushed hazelnut or sliced almonds for garnish
50 g raw cacao mass
50 g maple
A handful of mulberries for garnish

1. Melt the cacao butter in a double boiler with the lowest heat setting. The temperature should be around 107° F (42° C) to keep it in raw. Add the cacao mass and mix until everything combined well and smooth. Once mixed, add the maple and mix again mix until completely smooth and liquid.

2. Place a parchment paper into the pyrex or pan.

3. Pour the chocolate over the parchment.

4. Sprinkle crushed hazelnuts or sliced almonds, dried mulberries and quinoa pops.

5. Let it rest at least 30 minutes in room temperature.

6. Then Place into the refrigerator at least 3 hours before using.

SWEETS

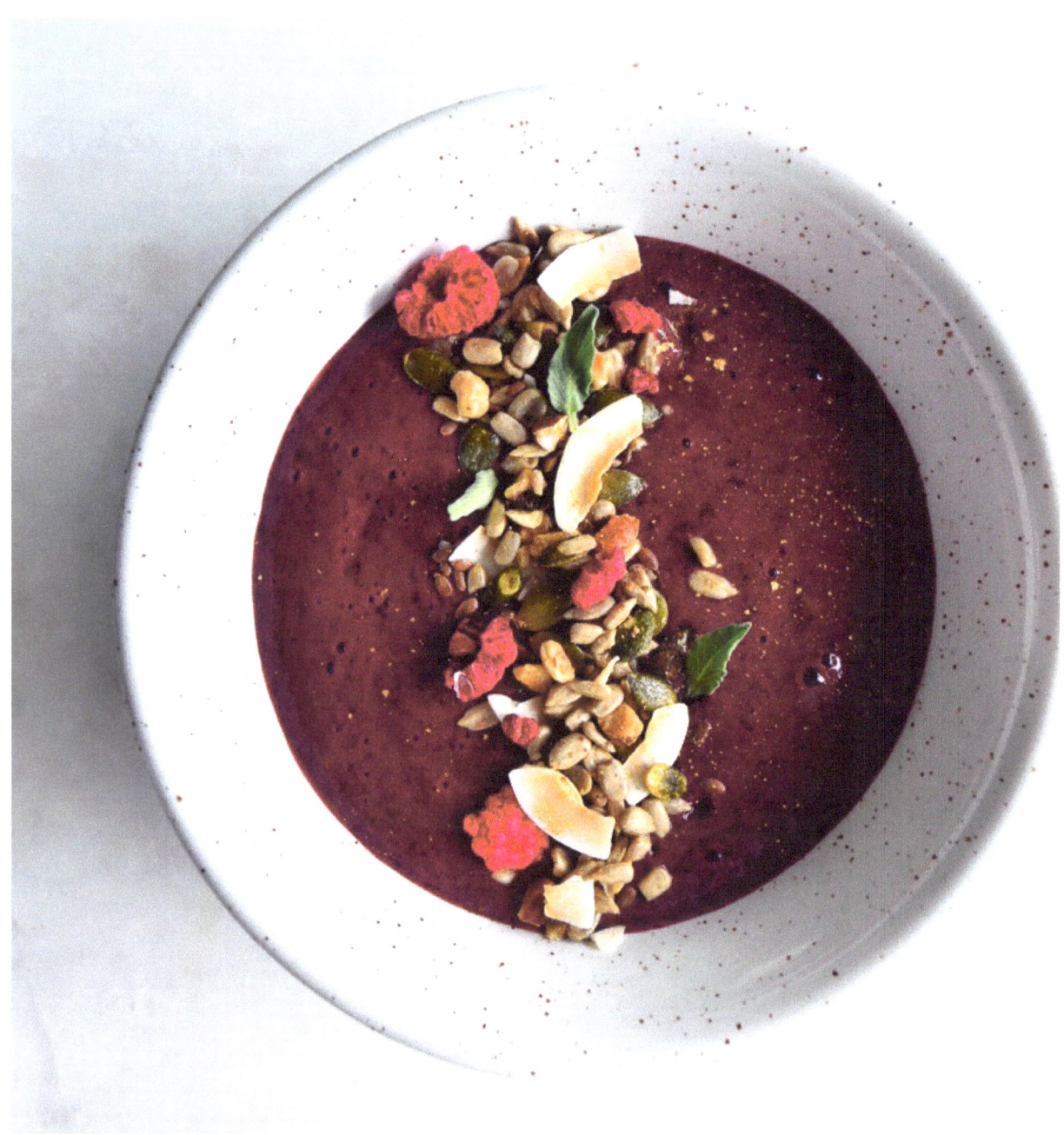

ACAI BOWL

Time - 10 minutes
Serves - 2

Ingredients
4 frozen bananas
1 cup frozen mixed berries
A handful of fresh spinach
1 tbsp tahini or nut butter
1 tsp maca powder
2 tbsp acai powder

Toppings
Pumpkin seeds, sunflower seeds, freeze dried raspberries, fresh sage leaves, coconut chips, chopped hazelnuts

1. Place all the ingredients except decoration ingredients in the blender and processn until completely smooth.
We want it thick and smooth, so avoid adding liquid.

2. Pour in your bowl, top with desired toppings.

3. Eat cold!

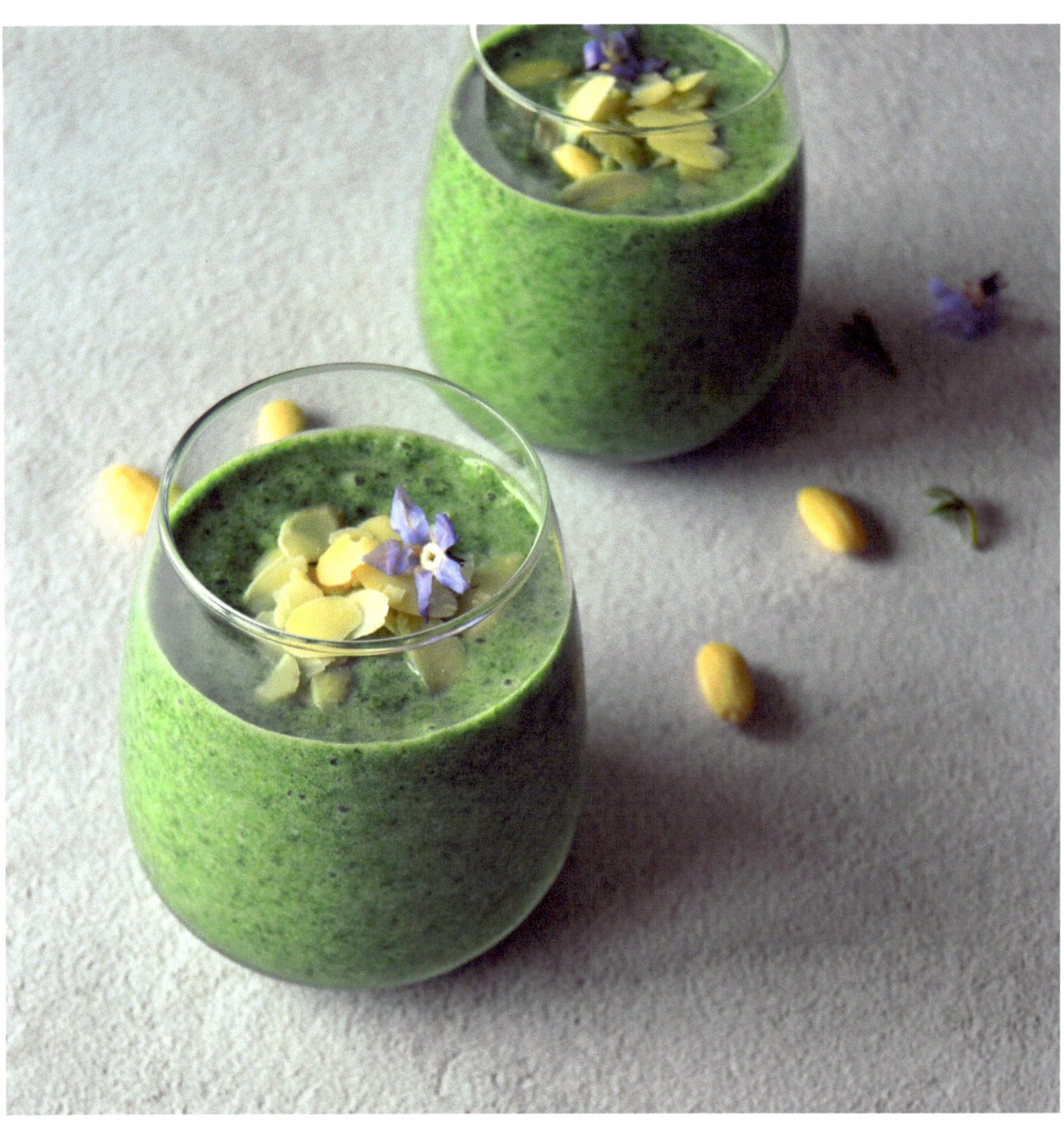

SPINACH BANANA SMOOTHIE

Time - 5 minutes
Serves - 2

Ingredients
3 ripe bananas
1 cup frozen spinach
1 cup almond milk
1 tsp spirulina
1 tbsp tahini or nut butter
3-4 dates or 1/4 cup mulberries
1/4 tsp nutmeg

Toppings
Borage leaves
Sliced almonds

1. Place the banana, spinach , dates, desired nut butter, and almond milk into the blender.

2. Mix on high speed until smooth. Add a pinch nutmeg and stir well.

3. Pour mixture into glasses.

4. Decorate with sliced almonds and star flower if desired. Enjoy cold!

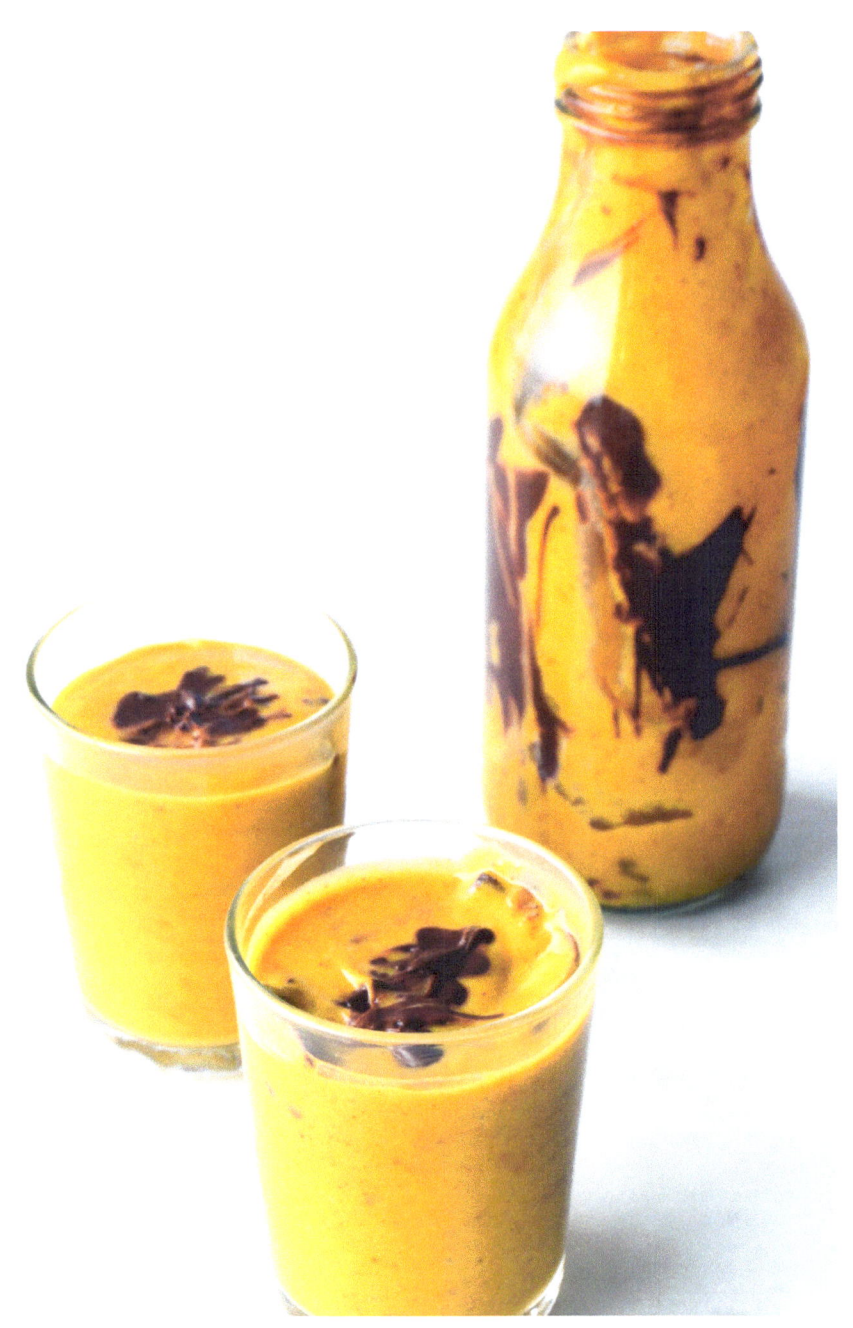

PUMPKIN SMOOTHIE

Time - 5 minutes
Serves - 2

Ingredients
130 g cooked pumpkin
200 g frozen banana
25 g almond butter
1 tbsp maple syrup
1/2 cup plant milk
1/4 tsp all spice
Raw dark chocolate optional to drizzle

1. Cut the pumpkin into small pieces and steam until soft. Let chill. Freeze pieces in the freezer until the next day or at least 3-4 hours. You can also use pumpkin raw if you prefer.

2. Blend all ingredients until smooth and creamy. Add maple and plant milk until the perfect consistency is reached. We love our smoothies thick and spoonable.

3. Melt raw dark chocolate and drizzle it inside the smoothie jars.

4. Pour smoothie mixture. Serve immediately.

INDEX

A

- ACAI BOWL 199
- ALFREDO SAUCE 123
- ALMOND BRITTLE 175
- ALMOND PINK CHEESE 15
- ARTICHOKE PEA SOUP 57
- ARTICHOKE WITH PEAS 43
- ARTICHOKE WITH PEAS, CARROT AND PINEAPPLES 33
- ASPARAGUS SOUP 51
- AVOCADO CHOCOLATE MOUSSE 194
- AVOCADO PITAYA CARPESE SALAD 93
- AVOCADO SAUCE 91

B

- BEETROOT PESTO 41
- BELUGA SALAD WITH SPINACH, BRUSSELS SPROUTS 63
- BIRCHER MUESLI 17
- BLACK BEAN SALAD WITH AVOCADO & PURSLANE 89
- BROAD BEAN SOUP 49
- BROWN RICE AND OKRA WITH PEAR CREAM 113
- BRUSSELS SPROUTS WITH POMEGRANATES & PECAN 87
- BRUSSELS SPROUTS, MASHED POTATO & AVOCADO 91
- BUCKWHEAT RISOTTO WITH MUSHROOMS 69
- BUDDHA BOWL 151

C

- CARPESE AVOCADO PITAYA SALAD 93
- CAULIFLOWER ALMOND GRATIN 96
- CAULIFLOWER LEEK SOUP 53
- CAULIFLOWER WITH PUMPKIN SAUCE 35
- CELERIAC CRUMB 125
- CELERIAC HASHBROWNS 37
- CELERIAC PAVE WITH CREAM AND CRUMB 125
- CELERIAC SALAD WITH APPLES AND SPINACH 61
- CHEDDAR SPREADABLE 13
- CHEESE FONDUE 16
- CHEESE MACADAMIA WITH SEAWEED 10
- CHEESE WITH ALMOND AND BEET 15
- CHICKPEA CURRY WITH CHANTERELLES 141
- CHICKPEAS WITH KALE 65
- CHILI CARROT QUINOA 71
- CHILI SAUCE 37
- CHIPOTLE BLACK BEANS 145
- CHOCOLATE MOUSSE WITH MULBERRY CRUMBLE 194
- CHOCOLATE MOUSSE WITH ALMOND BRITTLE 175
- CHOKLADBOLLAR - SWEDISH CHCOCOLATE BALLS 191
- CINNAMON BALLS 193
- COCKTAIL PIZZA BITES 18
- COCONUT BACON 29
- COCONUT OAT YOGURT 109
- COUSCOUS SALAD WITH CARROTS AND CASHEWS 77
- COWPEA SALAD WITH PROVENCE GREENS 83
- CRANBERRY PESTO 123
- CREAMY CEASAR SALAD WITH TEMPEH 111
- CROISSANT 165
- CRUNCHY EGGPLANTS 27

E

- EGGPLANTS OVEN BAKED 27

F

- FOCACCIA BREAD 23

G

- GARLIC CONFIT 50
- GINGER TAHINI DRESSING 101

H

- HABANERO SAUCE 133
- HALLONGROTTOR - SWEDISH STYLE RASPBERRY CAVES 161
- HEMP SEED CREAM 41

I

- ICELANDIC VINARTERTA 163
- IRISH POTATOES 21

J

- JACK IN WONDERLAND 129

K

- KALE WITH TOASTED CHICKPEAS 65
- KLADDKAKA - SWEDISH STYLE STICKY BROWNIE 155

L

- LINGON DONUT BALLS WITH MACADAMIA CREAM 159

M

- MACADAMIA CHEESE 10
- MAKING TEMPEH FROM SCRATCH 105
- MAPLE FRIED BRUSSELS SPROUTS 87
- MASHED POTATO WITH BRUSSELS SPROUTS 91
- MASHED PURPLE POTATO WITH MIXED MUSHROOMS 121
- MOONG DAL CHILLA IRISH POTATOES 45
- MULBERRY CRUMBLE 194
- MUNG BEAN WITH BLUEBERRIES 81

O

- OAT CHANTERELLE CREAM 117
- OAT COCONUT YOGURT 109
- OATMEAL 185
- OKRA, BROWN RICE WITH PEAR CREAM 113

P

- PASTA WITH ALFREDO & CRANBERRY PESTO 123
- PEAR WALNUT CRUMBLE 171
- PENNE WITH ALFREDO SAUCE AND BROCCOLI 149
- PHYLLO BÖREK 31
- PITAYA AVOCADO CARPESE SALAD 93
- PIZZA BITES 18
- PLUM TOMATO SAUCE 131
- PORCINI SOUP 55
- PORRIDGE WITH MUSHROOM & BERRIES 99
- PORTEBOLLO MUSHROOMS WITH SPINACH 25
- POTATO CURRY WITH KALE AND NUTS 143
- POTATO POCKETS 39
- POTATO SALAD WITH CHARD & BELUGA 101
- POTATOES IRISH STYLE 21
- POTATOES WITH BEET PESTO AND HEMP CREAM 41
- PROVENCAL COWPEA SALAD WITH KIWIS 83
- PULLED OYSTER MUSHROOMS 99
- PUMPKIN PIPETTE 135
- PUMPKIN SAUCE 35
- PUMPKIN SMOOTHIE 203

R

RASPBERRY PANNA COTTA 183
RAW BLUEBERRY COCONUT CHOCOLATE CAKE 189
RAW CAKE WITH FOREST FRUITS 187
RAW CHOCOLATE 197
RAW COFFEE CAKE 179
RAW OREOS 177
RAW SWEDISH PRINCESS CAKE 181
RAW VEGGIE SALAD WITH TAHINI DRESSING 85
RED CABBAGE SALAD 97
RED LENTIL DAHL WITH BUTTERNUT SQUASH CREAM 147
RICE WITH PEAS AND MALVA 67
RISOTTO BUCKWHEAT 69
RISOTTO WITH MUSHROOMS AND POMEGRANATES 139
ROASTED VEGGIE QUINOA SALAD 73

S

SAVORY PORRIDGE WITH MUSHROOM AND BERRIES 99
SEED CRACKERS 50
SEITAN FROM SCRATCH 137
SHEPHERD'S PIE WITH BELUGA 127
SPINACH BANANA SMOOTHIE 201
SUNCHOKES WITH SPINACH AND ASPARAGUS 95
SWEDISH ALMOND BREAD 167
SWEDISH ALMOND CAKE 169
SWEDISH CHOCOLATE BALLS 191
SWEDISH POTATO DUMPLINGS 115
SWEDISH PRINCESS CAKE 181
SWEDISH STYLE RASPBERRY CAVES 161
SWEDISH STYLE STICKY BROWNIE 155
SWEET POTATO CHOCOLATE CAKE 173

T

TABOULLEH BOWL 75
TAGLIATELLE WITH PLUM TOMATO SAUCE 131
TAHINI DRESSING 85
TEMPEH SATAY WITH SPICY HAZELNUT-GINGER SAUCE 119
TEMPEH WITH MUSHROOM COCONUT SAUCE & KALE 107
THREE LAYER FESTIVE RAW CAKE 157
TOFU WITH HABANERO SAUCE 133
TOSCATÅRTA - SWEDISH ALMOND CAKE 169

Q

QUINOA LENTIL SALAD WITH SHIITAKE 79
QUINOA WITH CHILI CARROT 71
QUINOA WITH ROASTED VEGGIES 73

V

VETELÄNGDER - SWEDISH ALMOND BREAD 167

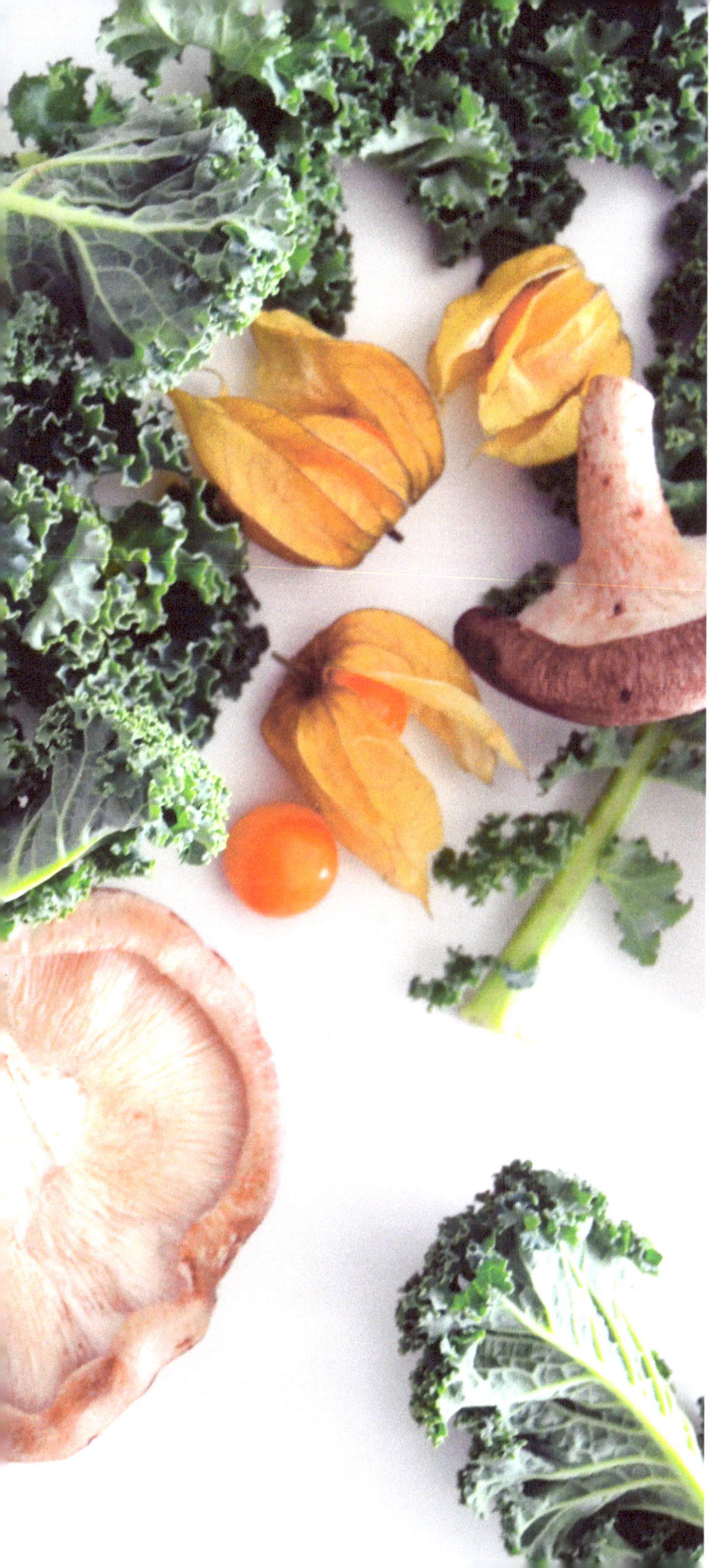

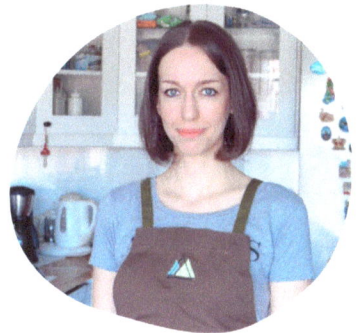

about the author

Nazlı Develi is a plant food designer, an inventive, aesthetically minded hands-on chef and artist with an eye for details and the founder of GREEN & AWAKE Plant Food Design Studio.

She specialized in plant based and raw cuisine, restaurant consultancy, recipe development, workshops, chef training and creative concepts, all rooted in food expression with nature as a core.

Obsessed with art, design, health, wellness and experimental flavours, she's strongly committed to spreading awareness about plant-based food as the most sustainable and necessary alternative for the planet.

Instagram: @gurmevegan
@greenandawake
Website: www.gurmevegan.com
www.greenandawake.com

www.ingramcontent.com/pod-product-compliance
Lightning Source LLC
Chambersburg PA
CBHW041706160426
43209CB00017B/1760